Essential Clinical Handbook for ENT Surgery

The ultimate companion for Ear, Nose and Throat surgery, including a chapter on facial plastic surgery

First edition

Edited by Dr. Desmond A. Nunez

Dr. John Bunni

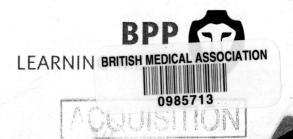

BPP

LEARNIN BRITISH MEDICAL ASSOCIATION

First edition 2013

ISBN 9781 4453 8169 5
e-ISBN 9781 4453 9394 0

British Library Cataloguing-in-Publication Data
A catalogue record for this book is available from the British Library

Published by
BPP Learning Media Ltd
BPP House, Aldine Place
London W12 8AA

www.bpp.com/health

Printed in the United Kingdom by Ricoh
Ricoh House
Ullswater Crescent
Coulsdon
CR5 2HR

Your learning materials, published by BPP Learning Media Ltd, are printed on paper sourced from sustainable, managed forests.

BPP
LEARNING MEDIA

Contents

2 Nose – rhinology

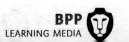

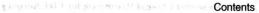
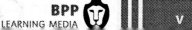

4   Facial plastic surgery

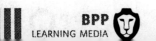

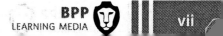

About the Publisher

BPP Learning Media is dedicated to supporting aspiring professionals with top quality learning material. BPP Learning Media's commitment to success is shown by our record of quality, innovation and market leadership in paper-based and e-learning materials. BPP Learning Media's study materials are written by professionally-qualified specialists who know from personal experience the importance of top quality materials for success.

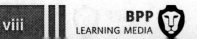

About the Authors

John Bunni, M.B., Ch.B(Hons), MRSC

Dr Bunni is a Specialist Registrar in General Surgery in Bristol. He completed his Basic Surgical Training in the South West of England, after graduating in Medicine from the University of Bristol with Honours in 2005. He subsequently completed his Membership Exams in 2008 and is in higher surgical training. He has an interest in laparoscopic colorectal surgery and has published several peer reviewed papers in General Surgery. He is an avid reader of the history of surgery and enjoys watching and playing tennis.

Desmond A. Nunez, MBBS MD FRCS(ORL)

Dr Nunez is Head of the Division of Otolaryngology, Full time faculty Associate Professor at the University of British Columbia in Vancouver Canada and Honorary Reader in Otolaryngology – Head & Neck Surgery at the University of Bristol, UK. He previously served as Director of the Department of Otolaryngology at North Bristol NHS Trust and led the University of Bristol MB Ch.B Otolaryngology programme until 2011. He was a member of the faculty of examiners of the Royal Colleges of Surgeons of Edinburgh, England, Glasgow and Ireland over the period from 2000–2011. Dr Nunez has over 90 publications in peer reviewed journals or text books and is an assistant editor of the *Journal of Laryngology and Otology*.

Mark J. Shikowitz, MD, MBA, FACS

Dr Mark Shikowitz is a member of the full-time academic faculty of the North Shore-LIJ Healthcare System. He has served as director of residency training, Associate Chairman, and now the Vice Chairman of the department. He is a full Professor of Otolaryngology at the Albert Einstein College of Medicine, Bronx, New York. His practice involves both adult and paediatric patients and has centred around nasal and sinus surgery, cosmetic facial and reconstructive surgery, and endoscopic skull base tumour surgery. Dr Shikowitz is the Director of the Zucker Nasal and Sinus Center which he helped to form. Dr Shikowitz has lectured and performed surgery around the world and published numerous peer reviewed articles and chapters in text books on related subjects.

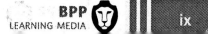

Acknowledgements

The authors acknowledge the support of colleagues Mr Farhan Ahsan, Mr Daniel Hajioff and Professor Hisham Khalil, who reviewed and commented on the text. The contributions of Dr David Pothier, Mr Andrew Carswell and Dr Rupert Ricks to the illustrations are likewise acknowledged.

Dr Mark Shikowitz was assisted by Anthony Joseph R. Santos, RPA-C. The artwork in Chapter 4 was produced by Wendy Beth Jackelow, MFA, CMI.

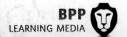

Preface

Most medical students' knowledge of rare diseases is good, due to a combination of rare cases being observed in specialist clinics or due to the fact that odd eponymous syndromes are much loved by examiners and hence added into most final medical school papers. However common symptoms are often not well taught or even considered relevant by many students and teachers alike – central retrosternal crushing pain ought to bear more weight that a runny nose, shouldn't it?

A significant proportion of medical students, 50% or more in the United Kingdom, will go on to become general practitioners, who will have no trouble with Felty's syndrome, phaeochromocytoma and McArdle's glycogen storage disease, yet will struggle with the differential diagnosis of a sore throat and its sequale based on their medical school teaching.

Thus this book has been designed with the intention of introducing today's medical student to what some may consider a postgraduate topic. It is designed to integrate diseases of the ears, nose and throat with all other areas of medicine. After all, the organism is the same and all organ systems interact together. It shows that ENT (Otolaryngology) and Head and Neck Surgery is not an isolated and unimportant/incomprehensible area of knowledge but an interesting and valuable area of medicine and surgery which is related to many other parts of the medical school curriculum.

Hence, a basic understanding of neurology, respiratory and emergency medicine is extremely important, as is all the relevant anatomy and physiology, to fully appreciate ENT.

With every applicable topic (ears, nose throat etc) there will be notes on 'What to do in an OSCE'; doubtless this will be the focus of most students. This book is intended as an introduction to ENT for whatever reason such as there not being enough ENT teaching, or books on the subject being too detailed and specialised, and also as a starting point to pick up key tips for OSCEs, clinics and future medical practice.

Finally, a lot of lists will be presented, to help you appreciate the key points.

John Bunni, M.B., Ch. B(Hons), MRSC

Desmond A. Nunez, MBBS MD FRCS(ORL)
Associate Professor and Head,
Division of Otolaryngology Head and Neck Surgery,
University of British Columbia,
Vancouver General Hospital, Vancouver Canada.
Honorary Reader in Otolaryngology,
Department of Clinical Sciences North Bristol,
University of Bristol, England

Mark J. Shikowitz, MD, MBA, FACS
Vice-Chairman, Department of Otolaryngology and Communicative Disorder
North Shore-LIJ Health System, New Hyde Park, NY, USA
Professor of Otolaryngology
The Albert Einstein School of Medicine, Bronx, NY, USA
Professor, Department of Otolaryngology
Hofstra North Shore-LIJ School of Medicine, Hempstead, NY, USA
Director, Zucker Nasal and Sinus Center,
North Shore-LIJ Health System, New Hyde Park, NY, USA

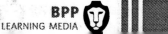

Foreword

Ear Nose and Throat education has never hit the headlines and features weakly in medical school curricula. After all, what can be more important than hearts, brains, lungs? What can be more exciting than emergency abdominal surgery and resuscitation? What can challenge our emotions more than sick children and cancer?

Yet ENT, as much medicine as it is surgery, is fundamentally about keeping people human. Hearing and speech mean that we can communicate like no other animals, they are the basis, even more than sight, of our interaction with the people around us, indeed of society, of our lives themselves.

In their preface, the authors of Essential Clinical Handbook for ENT, decorated scholars and teachers all, point out how despite the fact that up to 20% of primary care consultations and secondary care referrals are for ENT disorders, doctors all over the world leave medical school poorly equipped to deal with even the basics of this varied, engrossing specialty.

There are elements of paediatrics, cancer and emergency care here for those with traditional aspirations. But for those fledgling doctors wanting to affect the health of as many people as possible, and at the same time maintain the fabric of a healthy, communicative society, this book shows them how, through excellent ENT care. And it does it simply, effectively and with style.

Would that I had had it beside me before my own Finals....

Martin Birchall MA MD (Cantab) FRCS, F Med Sci
Professor of Laryngology, University College London
ENT Programme Director, UCL Partners Academic Health Science System
Consultant Otolaryngologist, Royal National Throat Nose and Ear Hospital, London, UK

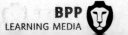

Chapter 1

Ears – otology

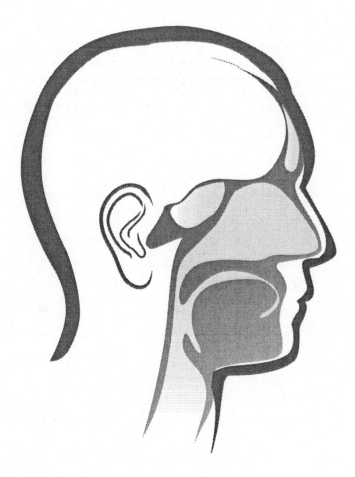

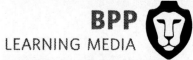

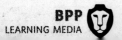

A brief outline of the relevant anatomy and physiology will be discussed so as to bridge pre-clinical science and clinical medicine. This will be followed by clinical history taking and examination in a succinct, easy-to-digest form.

Introduction

Hearing is one of our valuable senses. However, it must be borne in mind that although it is always thought that the ears are what hear, this is far too simplistic. It is in fact the brain that 'hears' and the ears are only a medium that channel and transduce sound waves (collision of air molecules) into action potentials that reach the auditory cortex in the temporal lobe. The fact that the brain is the organ of hearing is well illustrated by the story of Dmitri Shostakovich, the Soviet composer who as a result of a shell exploding near him in World War II could 'hear' music by tilting his head to one side. This was because the metal shell, when his head was tilted, came into contact with and activated his auditory cortex.

Anatomy and physiology of the ear and hearing

What is sound?

This is not only a scientific question but also a philosophical one, however the former only will be considered. As far as we know, sound waves are **propagated disturbances of particles in the medium conducting the sound**. This is the reason why in space 'no one can hear you scream', due to the vacuum that exists – there are no air molecules (on average one atom per metre squared exists) to collide and hence form what we call sound. The sound intensity is equal to the pressure change multiplied by the volume velocity. The human ear is sensitive to tones with frequencies between 20Hz to 20,000Hz. It is most sensitive to sounds between 2,000Hz and 5,000Hz. This will be discussed further in *Investigations*.

Hearing

To consider how hearing works it is necessary to appreciate the layout of the auditory system. It is divided into outer ear, middle ear and inner ear and a nervous pathway from the inner ear to the hindbrain (brainstem) and auditory cortex. To remind you of what the ear (auditory system) looks like see Figure 1.1.

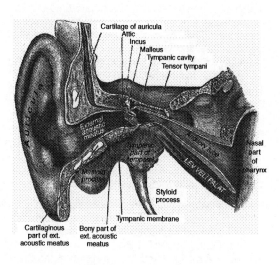

Figure 1.1 Coronal section displaying anatomical relationships of outer, middle and inner ear Gray H (1918) Anatomy of the Human Body, 20th edition, Lea & Febiger, Philadelphia
(This image is in the public domain because its copyright had expired. This applies worldwide.)

The external ear

The external ear consists of the pinna (auricle), external auditory meatus and auditory canal. The auditory canal is made up of an outer cartilaginous one-third and inner bony two-thirds. It is skin lined throughout but with sebaceous glands and hair follicles in the outer third only. The skin is thin, tightly adherent to the underlying bone and sensitive in the inner two-thirds. It ends at the tympanic membrane ('ear drum').

The middle ear

The middle ear consists of the tympanic membrane (TM) and a chain of auditory ossicles (bones – the smallest in the body incidentally) called the **malleus** (hammer), **incus** (anvil) and **stapes** (stirrup). It is the TM that separates the external ear from the middle ear. The oval window and round window separate the middle ear from the inner ear (shown above). The middle ear is air filled also. It is the middle ear and external ear that fulfil more of a mechanical function in terms of capturing and directing sound waves whereas the inner ear is where the sophisticated neurophysiology occurs.

Before sound is heard the alternating air pressure is directed into the auditory canal via the external ear (pinna) which transmits the sound onto the TM. This causes the TM to vibrate and this is carried down the chain of ossicles to the foot plate of the stapes in the oval window (the stapes has a footplate which inserts into the oval window and is the interface between middle ear and inner ear). The surface area of the foot plate is much less than the TM thus amplifying the pressure changes as well as the mechanical advantage of the lever system of ossicles. This minimises the attenuation (impedance) normally caused when sound waves move from a less dense medium to a more dense medium (picture yourself blowing a bubble under water – it's a lot harder than blowing into air).

If vibrations are too loud the evolutionary adaptation to this is contraction of the tensor tympani muscle on the malleus and stapedius on the stapes to reduce sound amplification. (This could be an end-of-year MCQ/asked by a surgeon in theatre – examiners love these questions!)

The inner ear

We are not going to go into too much detail here about potassium currents and endolymph, but it is important to understand some of the physiology to commonly distinguish between conductive and sensorineural hearing loss.

The inner ear consists of the cochlea which is concerned with hearing; the utricle, saccule and three semicircular canals (bony labyrinth) which detect directions in head movement. The cochlea consists of three canals. The upper and lower canals (scala vestibuli and tympani) are filled with perilymph and the middle canal (Scala Media) is filled with endolymph (similar to cerebrospinal fluid (CSF)). Inside the middle canal is the organ

of Corti. This contains the sensory hair cells (sound receptors) that depolarise on deformation transducing mechanical vibrations into a depolarising current for nerve transmission. All the afferent nerve fibres and their interconnections from the individual receptors join to form the auditory nerve which will conduct action potentials to the auditory cortex of the brain.

Thus once the oval window vibrates the perilymph in the scala vestibuli this transmits the vibrations to the endolymph in the Scala Media which stimulates the organ of Corti causing fluxes of electrolyte-generated currents resulting in auditory impulses being sent to the relevant part of auditory cortex.

The pathway is from the organ of Corti to afferent cochlear nerves which synapse with dorsal and ventral cochlear nuclei of the medulla which then ascend the CNS. These pathways are important as brain tumours may interrupt them and the patient may present with hearing loss. Problems from the pons/midbrain/temporal lobe can lead to hearing loss. They are the important parts if you are not interested in detail.

This is the basic physiology of hearing. To illustrate this further you will find some figures below with notes describing important learning points and tips.

Anatomy of the pinna and tympanic membrane

Below is a picture of the pinna. You should be able to recognise and name the lobule, the tragus and the helix.

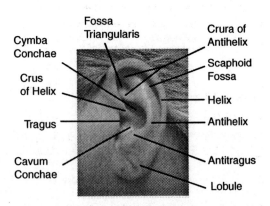

Figure 1.2 The anatomy of the adult pinna. (Reproduced with permission from Dr B Ghorayeb.)

Tympanic membrane (TM)

This will be discussed in more detail in the *Clinical examination* section. However, you ought to familiarise yourself with what the TM looks like and try to see as many as you can on the ward/ in clinic otherwise it will not make sense. Learn to recognise at least the attic, handle and umbo of the malleus (labelled Figure 1.3 below).

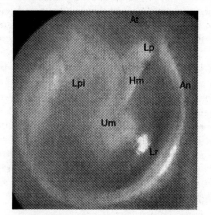

Figure 1.3 Annotated normal tympanic membrane.

Key:

An: *Annulus fibrosus*

Lpi: *Long process of incus* – sometimes visible through a healthy translucent drum

Um: *Umbo* – the end of the malleus handle and the centre of the drum

Lr: *Light reflex* – antero-inferioirly

Lp: *Lateral process of the malleus*

At: *Attic* also known as *pars flaccida*

Hm: *Handle of the malleus*

The ear and balance

Balance is maintained by many interactions of several systems including the cerebellum, reticular system, visual input, vestibular input and proprioceptive system. To appreciate vestibular causes of balance pathology an understanding of basic physiology is necessary.

Above the cochlea are three endolymph filled semicircular canals which are responsible for detecting angular/rotational head movement. These three semicircular canals are arranged at right angles to each other and thus can detect movement in all three physical planes. There are also otolith organs (utricle and saccule on the

medial wall of the vestibule) which respond to gravity and linear acceleration.

At the end of each canal there is a swelling (an ampulla), inside of which are sensory hair cells. The distal ends of the vibrissae (hairs) from these cells are embedded in a gelatinous mass called a cupula. The cupula spans the whole length of the ampulla and has the same specific gravity as the endolymph in the canal. Thus during angular acceleration of the head the cupula is displaced and therefore causes excitation or inhibition of the hair cells. When the head is displaced the semicircular canals move in the same direction, but the fluid inside will move in the opposite direction to that of the head movement and hence will displace the cupula and thus stimulate the hair cells. The nerve impulses generated pass along from the afferent vestibular nerve to the cerebellum and brain stem via the medial longitudinal fasciculus. It is in the cerebrum where head movement is perceived. Rotation leads to increased vestibular input from one side and reduced from the opposite side.

Vestibulo-ocular reflex

This is a reflex that is open looped and not regulated by feedback but is regulated by the cerebellum. It is a visual reflex that occurs as a response to head movement in one direction. If the head is rotated in one direction then initially the eyes move to the same degree in the opposite direction to maintain the direction of gaze.

The reflex is mediated through the connections between the vestibular brain stem nuclei and those controlling eye movement, namely the abducent and oculomotor, the latter via the medial longitudinal fasciculus. This results in changes in tone of the medial and lateral recti muscles; contracting one and relaxing the other (with the aid of vestibular nuclear input) such that the eyes are moved in the opposite direction to head movement.

This is important to understand because it explains the sensation of vertigo (discussed later). Briefly, vertigo (subjective sensation of movement,) occurs when there is a mismatch of sensory input. It is due to a conflict between vestibular and visual input ie your eyes and ears contradict each other in the information they tell you ('you' being your brain). For example, if you have suffered a bout of acute vestibular neuritis and have lost function of one peripheral vestibular system (eg a semicircular canal) then the mismatch between the ears will, through the action of the above reflex, move the eyes and induce a sensation of visual data moving – vertigo!

The above covers some of the basic science necessary to understand diseases of the ear and a lot can be worked out from first principles.

Clinical history

The history of a patient with an ear, nose or throat complaint like all other clinical histories is **the key to obtaining a diagnosis**. A good history is not easy to take, though it may appear so. It is not just about asking questions but relies on good listening skills including observing the patient's behaviour and features when providing a description of their complaints. Addressing the patient's worries and concerns allows them to leave the consultation feeling better. History taking skills must be practised and practised until you become more proficient in making an accurate diagnosis.

The main features to assess in the history of a patient with an otological complaint include:

- Hearing
- Tinnitus
- Balance (vertigo/dizziness)
- Ear discharge (otorrhoea)
- Ear pain (otalgia)

This list is not difficult to remember, and if you forget, just think about what the ear does (hearing and balance) and what can go wrong.

The following will each be looked at in detail but as part of the full history you should also ask about:

- Previous ear surgery (under PMH – previous medical history)

- Drug history (ototoxic drugs – frusemide, cardiac glycosides, antibiotics – streptomycin, gentamicin)

- Allergies (atopic disease)

- Family history (hearing loss etc)

- Occupation (noise exposure)

- Review of systems (systemic disease eg stroke, multiple sclerosis, the cardiovascular history is very important as is the neurological history for patients presenting with ear complaints. Don't forget eponymous syndromes associated with hearing loss eg Alport's.)

Otological symptoms

Hearing loss

Hearing loss is a very important symptom and can cause a great deal of worry and anxiety to the patient. The first thing to do is take a good history even though this may prove difficult. Ask about why they think they have a hearing problem: does their family say the TV is too loud, do they frequently have to ask others to repeat what has been said with their hand behind their ear? How long have they suffered a hearing deterioration? Was the loss sudden or gradual? If sudden it may be due to thromboembolism, if gradual it may be age associated or due to excessive noise exposure. Is there a history of ear infections? How does the hearing loss affect their life – do they work in a telesales centre or are they an 85-year-old recluse with angina? Not that you shouldn't try to treat the latter patient, but the benefits and risks of surgical interventions, if required, need to be properly assessed in all cases.

Hearing loss can be categorised into conductive or sensorineural hearing loss.

Conductive hearing loss

This is impaired sound transmission through the external ear canal and middle ear to the the oval window, ie it is a problem with the outer or middle ear. Thus anything that can go wrong in those spaces can cause a conductive hearing loss.

Common causes include:

- External canal obstruction due to wax, infection or foreign body

- Tympanic membrane perforation due to trauma, infection

- Otosclerosis (an overgrowth of the bone of the inner ear resulting in fixation of the stapes in the oval window, which leads to conductive hearing loss)

- Otitis media

- Ossicular chain discontinuity secondary to trauma or infection

The above pathologies will be dealt with in more detail so don't worry if you don't understand it all yet; just have a picture of what a conductive hearing loss is.

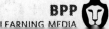

Sensorineural hearing loss

This is different to conductive in that the pathways of sound conduction to the inner ear are normal yet there is still hearing loss. This is due to pathology medial to the oval window (ie the inner ear) and this may be a problem with the cochlea, cochlear nerve or even the central auditory pathways (ie midbrain problems etc).

Conductive and sensorineural hearing loss are usually easy to distinguish from one another on examination, yet history-wise all the other ear questions should be asked, for example, ear discharge, as this may give you a clue as to the underlying cause.

Common causes include:

* Presbyacusis (age-related hearing loss due to gradual loss of cochlear hair cells)

* Infections (meningitis, measles, mumps, cytomegalovirus, toxoplasmosis, other causes of bacterial labyrinthitis)

* Congenital (syndromic and nonsyndromic hearing losses)

* Ototoxic drugs (see above)

* Ménière's disease

* Trauma

* Cerebrovascular disease (a stroke or temporary ischaemic attack can present with or be associated with loss of hearing)

Less common causes but important:

* Tumour – acoustic neuroma (benign tumour of vestibular nerve sheath)

* Medical conditions in which a proportion of patients develop sensorineural hearing loss (rare causes of hearing loss)

* Multiple sclerosis

* Hypothyroidism

* Sarcoidosis

Try to remember the first three from the common causes list and the first from the less common causes list.

The impact of the hearing loss on the patient, their family, friends and employment prospects should be assessed. A history obtained from an accompanying partner or family member may help in this regard. In what listening situations does the patient experience a hearing problem (on the phone, in shops, in background noise etc)? Has the patient given up a pastime, lost their job or avoids certain situations since the hearing loss developed?

Tinnitus

Tinnitus is not just ringing or buzzing in the ear but the sensation of any noise in the ear or even head. The sound is usually high pitched, so do ask about pitch. Ask **when** the tinnitus started, if they have had any head **trauma**, if they suffer from an **affective disorder** (eg depression) and if so if it came on before or after the tinnitus. Also determine if they suffer from **epilepsy** or even schizophrenia (but do be tactful). A history of noise exposure, anaemia, hypertension and drug use (prescribed and illicit) should be explored. Family history and stress are also important. As with pain ask about character, exacerbating and alleviating factors. Can anyone else hear the ringing? Is the tinnitus episodic and if so how long do the attacks last?

Bear in mind that tinnitus is common. 10 to 15% of the population in the UK and the USA seek medical attention because of tinnitus, 0.5–2% are severely affected. The prevalence increases with age. The aetiology in most cases is not known. Proposed mechanisms include increased activity in the peripheral auditory pathway such as outer hair cell generated spontaneous otoacoustic emissions and 'cross-talk' between adjacent nerve fibres in the central auditory pathway. Regardless, common causes should be excluded.

Common causes include:

* Wax
* Noise
* Ménière's disease
* Presbyacusis
* Ototoxic drugs

The importance of psychogenic factors such as emotional stress in triggering tinnitus is not to be underestimated. Symptoms usually increase at night perhaps due to the quiet, and this can interfere with the patient's sleep.

The tinnitus red flags are unilateral, objective (tinnitus that can be heard by an observer) and pulsatile tinnitus. Unilateral tinnitus may be a feature of an acoustic neuroma, objective and pulsatile tinnitus are suggestive of a vascular anomaly or glomus tumour respectively.

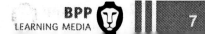

The treatment consists of whole person care and treating the cause. Reassurance is very important, especially if the patients are emotionally vulnerable; telling them that there is no sinister cause is often enough. Behavioural therapies such as tinnitus retraining therapy have high success rates. Usually, tinnitus does get better with time which is encouraging.

Pain (otalgia)

First things first, find out about the:

- Site
- Onset
- Character
- Radiation
- Alleviating factors
- Exacerbating factors
- Timing of pain (am versus pm)
- Severity
- Associated factors, eg nausea, vomiting etc

Primary otalgia common causes include:

- Otitis externa

- Otitis media (acute or with an effusion)

- Foreign body in external ear canal (beware the button battery placed by a child in the ear canal)

- Impaction of wax

Less common important causes:

- Neoplasia of the ear
- Mastoiditis

An important cause of otalgia is mastoiditis, inflammation of the mastoid cavity and cells. It is usually an extension of middle ear disease. It commonly presents with headache, pain over the mastoid bone (part of the temporal bone behind the ear), fever and hearing loss. Mastoiditis in the Western world most commonly presents in children as a complication of acute otitis media and is comparatively rare. Treatment is conservative, medical or surgical. Always treat the underlying cause, as well as administering systemic and/or topical analgesics.

Always remember referred pain. There are five nerves that refer pain to the ear and these are important. The non-otological areas supplied by these nerves should be examined when assessing a patient with otalgia. The nerves and potential conditions affecting them are as follows:

Auricular branch of CN V	→ Sphenoid sinus, teeth, temporomandibular joint
Greater auricular nerve (C2, 3)	→ Neck wound, cervical disc disease, osteoarthritis
Sensory branch of CN VII	→ Geniculate herpes (Ramsay Hunt syndrome)
Tympanic branch of CN IX and auricular branch of CN X	→ Throat eg tonsillitis, laryngeal cancer

Bear in mind that temporomandibular disorder pain is more commonly related to problems with the jaw muscles (myofacial pain) than with the temporomandibular joint (TMJ) itself. Ask about jaw noises, if it clicks, restricted jaw opening, teeth clenching and bruxism. Finally, neurological causes must be asked about, eg migraine, neuralgias etc – it will be obvious from the history, for example trigeminal neuralgia (eg intense stabbing pain in the trigeminal nerve region – remember ophthalmic, maxillary and mandibular divisions). If no pathology is found within the ear itself, then it is especially important that causes for referred otalgia be explored and excluded.

Discharge (otorrhoea)

Otorrhoea is very unpleasant, not only for the patient, but for those around them. Thus on questioning, the patient must **not** at all be made to feel uncomfortable or embarrassed. Enquire about the duration, what colour the discharge is, what the smell is like, if they have had it before.

If it is clear it could be cerebrospinal fluid (CSF). If it is coloured yellow/green it may be an infection (usually green is pseudomonas). The presence of mucus suggests a middle ear origin. Is there any blood coming from the ear? Haematorrhoea may be due to:

- Ear canal or tympanic membrane trauma

- Fractured base of skull (not difficult to identify from history of head trauma)

- Malignancy

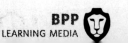

Facial nerve function is important, and some of the pathologies that cause otorrhoea (discussed below) can affect the nerve's function. Patients are acutely aware of a change in facial nerve function and will volunteer symptoms of dysfunction spontaneously including facial asymmetry, difficulty in eye closure and inadequate lip seal leading to drooling of saliva. Clinical examination of facial nerve function is described later in the text.

The common causes of otorrhoea are:

If less than six weeks' duration:

- Otitis externa
- Acute otitis media with TM perforation

If greater than six weeks' duration:

- Chronic Otitis Media (COM)
- Foreign body
- Neoplasia
- Necrotising otitis externa which is associated with bone destruction

Treatment depends upon the cause.

Vertigo/dizziness

Vertigo, as mentioned earlier, is an illusion of movement. The first question to ask is what does the patient mean by dizziness? It is useful to spend some time working this out because classically a peripheral vestibular or neurological cause accounts for symptoms of vertigo or imbalance but will not be responsible for symptoms of syncope or near syncope. The term dizziness encompasses all of these symptoms. Other important questions are symptom duration, frequency, associated features related to the ear eg otorrohea, hearing loss, aural pressure (feeling of pressure in the ear) and tinnitus. Also ask about recent infections, medications and nystagmus (do your eyes flick quickly from side to side when you feel dizzy? This is usually commented on by observers).

Non-otological (ear) causes of dizziness are common and can often be identified from the history. Symptoms related to a non-otological aetiology include palpitations, tremor, sweating and loss of consciousness.

First the causes of vertigo will be noted and then the time course of each disease as this helps to clinch the diagnosis.

Common causes of vertigo:

Otological

- Benign Paroxysmal Positional Vertigo (BPPV)
- Acute vestibular neuritis
- Recurrent vestibulopathy
- Ménière's disease

Neurological

- Migraine
- Brain infarction
- Neuropathy (autonomic or peripheral eg in diabetes)
- Brain tumour
- Benign paroxysmal vertigo of childhood (not to be confused with BPPV above)
- Multiple sclerosis

General

- Postural hypotension
- Anaemia
- Musculoskeletal (proprioceptive dysfunction)
- Diabetes (hypoglycaemia)

Again, try to remember two or three causes from each list.

Symptoms	Probable diagnosis
Episodic vertigo lasting seconds/minutes related to head movements.	(BPPV)
Episodic vertigo spontaneous onset with hearing loss (sensorineural), tinnitus, headache, sensation of the ear being 'full', nausea and vomiting. Duration: 20 minutes to 24 hours.	Ménière's disease
Incapacitating vertigo requiring complete bed rest for 3–7 days. Symptoms gradually resolve with a return to normal after a few weeks.	Vestibular neuritis. Idiopathic vestibular failure/ischaemia.

Table 1.1 Descriptions of symptoms of some common otological causes of vertigo; note the differences in duration of vertigo.

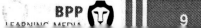

Treatment can be conservative, medical or surgical. Always treat the underlying cause. Treatments depend on the cause and vary from outpatient treatments such as the particle repositioning maneouvre (Epely) for BPPV to surgical division of the vestibular nerve for Ménière's disease.

We have now reached the end of quite a long section on clinical history. However it is probably the most important area to cover in depth within this text, as clinical examination is a skill best acquired through practice on the wards and in the clinics.

Clinical examination

Examination of the auditory system is not difficult with a routine, ordered approach.

The sequence for ear examination should be:

1. Introduction and permission to examine
2. Query tenderness/pain
3. Inspection
4. Otoscopic examination
5. Basic clinical tests of hearing
6. Rinne's test, Weber's test
7. Cranial nerves

Introduction and permission should be obvious, give your name, position, determine the patient's name, check in a clinical context if it corresponds with the case record notes and ask for consent to examine. Always ask about pain, as hurting the patient is the last thing that you ever want to do.

Inspection

This is just as important in the examination of the ear and the rest of the otolaryngology examination as it is in general medicine or surgery. A lot of valuable information can be gathered from a full inspection. Usually, medical students have a habit of a swift look, stating a memorised list of things to say regardless of whether they are there or not eg no scars, swelling, erythema etc. **Always** do a full inspection (if not for any other reason, it at least buys you time to think of what to do next!). Look for the following:

- External ear – size and shape of the pinna. Mention a few names eg no abnormality of the tragus and other anatomical structures shown in Figure 1.2.
- Look for extra cartilage and sinuses (an opening on the skin surface leading to a closed cavity) or pits.

- Evidence of trauma
- Skin lesions
- Discharge (appearance and **smell** – but be polite in describing the smell eg unpleasant not foul)
- Look for **scars**, in front of and behind the ears (pre- and post-auricular). You can use the light of the otoscope if you like, to aid your vision.
- Look at and palpate the mastoid bone for erythema and tenderness respectively. Is there evidence of inflammation (mastoiditis)? People commonly forget this.

Otoscopic examination

Practice is the key to getting to grips with the otoscope. Most people find it easier to use than the ophthalmoscope, probably because you don't have to fiddle with a magnifying lens and you are going into a canal to see rather than look at something straight ahead. Either way, practice makes perfect, or rather practice helps you to pass clinical skills assessment examinations.

Ensure that you know how to hold and switch on the otoscope. Check that the light is powerful by shining it on your hand. Fit one of the aural speculae (ends) onto the otoscope and try to pick the largest size that can comfortably fit into the ear but obviously not too big.

In adults you should hold the pinna with the thumb and forefinger of the hand not being used to hold the otoscope and pull it posteriorly and superiorly. This straightens the otherwise sigmoid shaped ear canal to allow the TM to be more clearly seen. This is why asking about pain is important at the start; you don't want to tug on someone's ear if it is very painful. Please also observe the patient when undertaking this manoeuvre for non verbal cues of discomfort. In children, you should only pull on the ear posteriorly and **not** superiorly, due to differences in anatomy.

Hold the otoscope in the hand corresponding to the ear you are examining, ie your right hand for the patient's right ear and vice versa. Grip the otoscope as you would hold a pen with your thumb, fore and middle fingers and bring your ring, little finger and ulnar border of your palm to rest on the patient's cheek as you would on a page you were writing on. Commonly first and even more advanced clinical year students are mortified at the idea of touching the patient's face when using the otoscope however be assured that this is best practice (despite the hammer grip popularised by many). This grip provides valuable tactile feedback

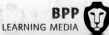

to the hand holding the otoscope while your eyes and brain are engaged in searching for the salient visual findings in the ear canal. If the patient flinches or moves their head abruptly you will be immediately alerted and it reduces the chance of traumatising the ear canal with the speculum as the hand holding the otoscope will mirror the head movement. In addition the bridge provided by your ring, little finger and ulnar border of your palm will prevent you over-inserting the otoscope into the ear canal (a common pitfall for the novice otoscopist!). Practise this.

When you are inside, there are several important points:

- The view obtained through the distal end of the otoscopic speculum at any one time is not usually comprehensive (do not expect to see the otoscopic views portrayed in this and other texts when you first insert the otoscope. These images are traditionally captured with a rod lens telescope inserted into the ear canal).

- Adopt a methodical approach to ensure that you see all of the ear canal and not only the tympanic membrane (medical students frequently make the mistake of overlooking the ear canal). Make a determined effort to see the anterior, superior, posterior and inferior walls of the ear canal, before going onto look at the tympanic membrane.

You may be able to practise on plastic models of the ear but the best way is to practise on humans, if your friends are willing to lend you their ears!

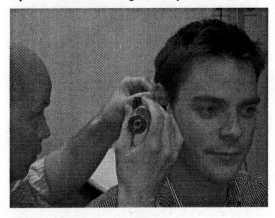

Figure 1.4 How to hold the otoscope.
(Library property of DA Nunez)

What to look for

Look at the state of the canal, is there any wax? Is there so much that it is obstructing your view? Any foreign bodies, bleeding, discharge, masses, defects, oedema? What is the colour, lucency and state of the TM? Is it retracted, protruberant or perforated? A knowledge of the normal anatomy of the TM is very important. Look at Figure 1.3 for a view of the normal TM.

You should be able to identify the lateral process of the malleus, the cone of light and the pars tensa and pars flaccida (attic). Note the lateral process of the malleus points anteriorly and thus if ever you have a data interpretation OSCE which includes images of tympanic membranes you can quickly work out which relates to the left and right ear by checking where the lateral process points: up and left, it is the left ear, and up and right, the right ear.

Occasionally, in a translucent TM you can see the long process of the incus and chorda tympani nerve. However it is more important to characterise the appearance of the ear drum. Is it red, is there a perforation? Figure 1.3 will help you gain a better insight into some abnormal tympanic membranes.

Clinical tests of hearing

Basically, you can mask the ear that is not being tested by massaging the tragus (the cartilage structure in front of the ear canal) into the conchal bowl with your index finger. Alternatively you can instruct the patient to undertake this manoeuvre. Additionally shield the patient's eyes to ensure that they do not speech read the movements of your lips. Say different numbers into their test ear and ask them to repeat them. Start off at a speech level that you are confident the patient can hear just to check that they are following your instructions and repeating the words/numbers you are saying. Once this is confirmed alter the volume of your speech, testing their responsiveness with a whisper, quiet speech, loud speech etc. Start at an arm's length (60cm/2 feet) away and then if they can't hear move to ear level (15cm/6 inches). Obviously stop if they can hear the quieter sounds at 60cm!

Normal hearing people should be able to hear a whisper presented at arm's length from the ear.

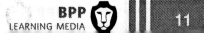

Rinne and Weber's tests

You may already know this from your neurology attachment, if not, don't worry. The point of these tests is that they can differentiate between a conductive and a sensorineural hearing loss and are thus very useful. They are both tuning fork tests ideally performed with a **512Hz** or **256Hz** tuning fork. It is impossible to interpret these tests without prior knowledge of the patient's hearing ability so do not use them to determine if the patient has a hearing loss. A clinical voice test will tell you if the patient has a hearing loss.

Rinne's test

Rinne's test is used to detect a conductive hearing loss. Hold the tuning fork at the base (the coin shaped bit at the end, if you have this design available) and strike the prongs on your elbow, knee or palm of hand but not on the furniture or your shoes (not too hard) to make it vibrate. Explain to the patient what you are about to do and do the following.

After achieving a vibrating tuning fork, place the prongs next to the patient's ear, at about 6cm (2.5 inches) away (with the parallel flat surfaces, not the tips, of the two prongs parallel to the external ear canal to maximise sound transmission) before placing the base of the tuning fork on the mastoid bone (behind the ear), remembering to stabilise the patient's head with your other hand. It is normal for the patient to withdraw slightly from the cold metal of the tuning fork thus reducing sound transmission and the reliability of the test (see Figure 1.5). While it is ringing ask whether the patient hears it better near their ear or on the mastoid. Now, what ought to normally happen is that the patient should hear it louder near the ear because air conduction is better than bone conduction. However, if they have a conductive hearing loss due, for example, to too much wax (cerumen) then they will hear the sound better on their mastoid bone, as you have effectively bypassed the obstruction.

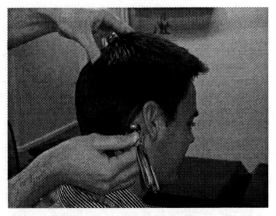

Figure 1.5 Rinne tunning fork test with the vibrating tuning fork placed on the patient's mastoid bone. Note the examiner's other hand is helping to stabilise the patient's head. (Library property of DA Nunez)

A normal Rinne, ie better hearing for sound presented by air, is termed Rinne positive (one of the tests where positive is normal). Recording the findings as air conduction greater than bone conduction or vice versa avoids this confusion and is better practice as your findings are recorded rather than an interpretation of the same. A false negative Rinne describes the findings of bone conduction better than air conduction in an ear with profound sensorineural hearing loss. This occurs because the air conduction stimulus cannot be perceived in the test ear and when the tuning fork is placed on the mastoid the sound is transmitted through the skull to the contra-lateral cochlea where it is perceived. The patient therefore reports hearing bone conduction better than air conduction.

You may think that's all there is too it, but the Rinne test will not give you the whole picture. What if there is a sensorineural loss without a conductive component? Air and bone conduction will both be reduced. The Rinne response will be identical to that of a patient without any hearing loss. That is why you ought to do the clinical tests of hearing first, to determine if there is a hearing loss at all before embarking on tuning fork tests.

Weber's test

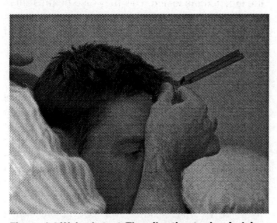

Figure 1.6 Weber's test. The vibrating tuning fork is placed on the patient's forehead. (Library property of DA Nunez)

Same drill, vibrate the tuning fork and this time place it on the patient's forehead in the midline (see Figure 1.6). The midline of the nasal bones or the vertex of skull are alternative positions. Ask the patient where they hear the sound better. It should be equal on both sides. If there is a sensorineural hearing loss, then the sound will be heard better in the **other** ear. If it is conductive it is heard better in the bad ear. This is quite difficult to grasp initially. Read the above again to ensure you fully understand.

Sensorineural → Heard better in **other** ear

Conductive → Heard better in **that** (bad) ear

So if you do Weber's test and the patient says they hear it better on their right ear, they could have left sensorineural hearing loss or right conductive loss (as the sound is transmitted through bone). So, do Rinne's test on their right ear, and if it is negative (ie better on mastoid) then you know they have a right conductive hearing loss. If Rinne is normal (ie positive) then they have a left sensorineural hearing loss.

Note. This only works if there is a unilateral hearing problem and like all tests there is a false negative and positive rate.

One final example is that if someone comes in with a **right sensorineural hearing** loss then they will have the following (see Table 1.2):

Tuning fork test	Right ear	Left ear
Rinne	Positive	Positive as normal air conduction
Weber		Sound localises here

Table 1.2 Tuning fork responses in a patient with a right sensorineural hearing loss

You should now be confident on differentiating the two types of hearing loss and remember some of the causes.

Conductive:

- Wax
- Infection

Sensorineural:

- Age related
- Noise trauma
- Infection
- Ménière's disease

Cranial and peripheral nerve examination

You should be able to undertake an examination of any of the cranial nerves especially the last nine which can be affected by ear disease. In addition review your tests of cerebellar function and lower limb touch and vibration sensation. The facial nerve examination is outlined below.

To tests its function, ask the patient to:

- Raise their eyebrows
- Show their teeth (smile)
- Puff out their cheeks

Remember that the forehead has bilateral representation in the brain and that in upper motor neurone lesions only the lower two-thirds is affected. However in lower motor neurone (LMN) lesions, all of one side of the face is affected. Bell's phenomenon may also be observed on asking the patient with a LMN lesion to close their eyes, ie the side affected won't be able to close, and the eye will go upwards and outwards while they try. The nerve to stapedius can be damaged and result in hyperacusis – undue sensitivity to sound. This can happen in disease of the seventh nerve eg Bell's palsy.

Neuro-otological examination

There are also special neuro-otological clinical tests to be undertaken when assessing the dizzy patient. These include:

- Romberg's test
- Head thrust (Halmagyi)
- Unterberger's (Fukuda) stepping test
- Dix-Hallpike's test

Romberg's test

If there is a proprioceptive or vestibular deficit, Romberg's test detects it. Romberg's does **not specifically** test cerebellar function (that is DANISH: **d**ysdiadochokinesis, **a**taxia, **n**ystagmus, **i**ntention tremor, **s**lurred/staccato speech and **h**ypotonia). Ask the patient to stand with feet together and eyes open initially. Then stand behind them and ask them to close their eyes. If there is a proprioceptive/vestibular defect their balance deteriorates and they **may** fall. The reason being that if there is a lesion in either the vestibular or proprioceptive system the patient compensates with the unaffected system and the visual system (eyes open). If visual information is also lost then so will balance as two of the three systems providing balance sensory input are non-functional.

Halmagyi head thrust

This is a test for unilateral vestibular weakness based on the vestibular ocular reflex. In brief hold the patient's head between the palms of your both hands. Request the patient to keep their eyes focused on an object in the mid-distance throughout the test. Then start by slowly rotating the patient's head alternately to the left and right. Observe the eyes for changes in gaze position. Then rotate the head rapidly to either side. If the eye movement to maintain gaze is delayed relative to your rotation of the head then the test is positive for weakness of the vestibular system on the side that you have rotated the head.

Fukuda (Unterberger's) stepping test

This is used to identify which labyrinth is not working in peripheral vertigo. Ask the patient to stand and march on the spot for 60 seconds with their eyes closed. If they start rotating to one side then the test is positive and the side rotated to is the side of the labyrinthine lesion. This may also be present in posterior fossa tumours (though other symptoms from the history are likely to be suggestive), and other central nervous system lesions.

Dix-Hallpike's test

This is the diagnostic test for Benign Paroxysmal Positional Vertigo. Place the patient sitting upright on an examination couch, with free space at the head end to allow you to support their head in your hands beyond the end of the couch. You should stand to one side of the couch facing the patient. Check that the patient has a full range of neck mobility before proceeding. Turn the patient's head 45 degrees to face the side of the couch you are standing next to (left or right). Then flex the patient's head 30 degrees from the vertical on the neck again to the side you are standing (left or right). Ask the patient to keep their eyes open and report if they experience vertigo. Now lower the patient swiftly to the supine position while maintaining their head's position relative to the body so that the head is supported 30 degrees below the level of the couch and is rotated 45 degrees to the left or right. Look for nystagmus (the chance of picking this up is improved if the patient's optic fixation is suppressed and the eyes magnifed with spectacles designed for this purpose). Wait for two to five minutes as the onset of nystagmus can be delayed and allow it to settle before continuing. Then return the patient to the sitting position and see if nystagmus returns. The classical positive response is the onset of rotatory nystagmus towards the underlying ear, the feature of BPPV arising from the posterior semicircular canal of the underlying ear. Repeat the manoeuvre to test the opposite side as the condition can be uni- or bilateral.

Naturally, you may want to check the blood pressure to exclude postural hypotension, check the pulse and auscultate the heart to look for cardiac causes of dizziness (arrhythmia, valvular heart disease, etc).

We will now look at several common pathologies, most of which have been mentioned already. They will be subdivided into diseases of the outer, middle and inner ear.

BPP LEARNING MEDIA

Investigations

The otological investigations that we will discuss are audiometry and tympanometry. Just like the ECG, you can figure a lot of it out from first principles.

Pure tone audiometry

This assesses hearing loss by air and bone conduction more accurately than Rinne's test. Basically sounds with a frequency between 125Hz and 8kHz are played to the patient either via earphones (air conduction) or a probe on the mastoid bone (bone conduction).

The intensity (amplitude) required for a particular frequency to be heard is plotted on an audiogram (graph of sound amplitude in dB (y axis) versus frequency in cycles per second (x axis).

The symbols used are:

Air conduction

Right   o
Left   x

Bone conduction (masked)

Right   [
Left   ]

When trying to grasp which masked bone conduction symbol refers to which ear, imagine the patient is facing you with head phones on both ears and each bracket symbol represents the headphone on the corresponding ear as follows: [0]. Therefore symbol ']' refers to the left ear.

Look at the position of the patient's plotted responses with respect to the horizontal line at 20dB. Normal hearing responses are at 20dB or better. Determine if there is a problem with the air and/or bone conduction. Is the problem at high frequencies (as in presbyacusis) or low frequencies? Below is an illustration of a patient's audiogram. Can you work out where the problem lies?

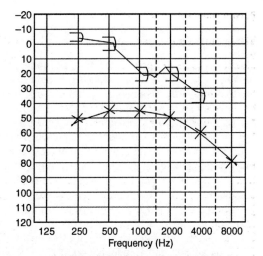

Figure 1.7 Audiogram showing air and bone conduction responses for the left ear. (Library property of DA Nunez)

This audiogram shows a left sided reduction in air and bone conduction leading to sensorineural loss, more so at high frequencies. If the right shows the same the diagnosis may be presbyacusis, if not and the right is fine, it may be an acoustic neuroma.

Impedance audiometry

The aim of impedance audiometry is to determine the state of the TM and the middle ear, and it aids the diagnosis of conductive hearing loss. This is achieved via tympanometry. This relies on the idea that when sound waves pass down the ear canal some will be absorbed by the ear and dissipated in making the TM vibrate, but some will also be reflected out of the ear canal. A taut TM reflects the most sound (just like a well made traditional drum). It is maximal when middle ear pressure equals atmospheric pressure. There are causes of a fall in middle ear pressure eg a blocked Eustachian tube (ET) or glue ear that reduce this impedance.

The data is plotted on a graph showing the amount of sound reflected by the middle ear (on the y axis) versus pressure in the external auditory meatus in deca Pascals (daPa) (on the x axis). The latter is altered by the tympanometer during the recording. The graph ought normally to be a bell with the peak at 0daPa. In pathology where the middle ear pressure is low (eg ET blockage) then the curve will shift to the left, because the pressure is lower (hence a left shift in the middle ear pressure measured on the x axis).

If very little sound is reflected then obviously the peak will be lower and the whole graph will be flatter. This is the case in glue ear.

How it works relies upon the fact that, as mentioned earlier, when the ear (either one) is subject to very loud sounds, the stapedius muscles of **both** ears contract so as to prevent damage. Now, normally this happens at about 75 decibels (dB). Thus if there is a hearing loss of 10dB then this reflex will kick in at 85dB and so forth. Thus, when you find out when the stapedius reflex is initiated, just subtract 75db from the figure and you will have your hearing loss calculated in dB. The impedance audiometer can tell when the reflex kicks in because the sudden contraction causes a reduction in sound absorbed by the middle ear (due to stiffening the ossicles) and thus an increase in reflected sound.

There are however certain contraindications for tympanometry. These are:

- Recently repaired TM
- Wax obstructing ear canal
- Oedema/damage of ear canal

Below are some results to illustrate what has been discussed.

ECV: 0.7 cm3   PEAK: 0.4 cm3
GR: 55 daPa   − 25 daPa   L

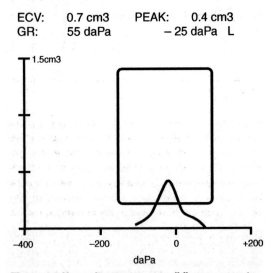

Figure 1.8 Normal tympanogram. (Library property of DA Nunez)

Ossicular restriction shows normal middle ear pressure, but reduced compliance. This could thus be due to a mechanical failure of the ossicles eg otosclerosis (stapes fixed to oval window leading to conductive hearing loss).

ECV: 0.6 cm3   PEAK: 0.2 cm3
GR: 155 daPa   − 95 daPa   R

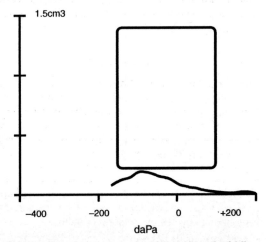

Figure 1.9 Tympanogram showing reduced middle ear compliance. (Library property of DA Nunez)

There are a number of other audiometric and vestibular function investigations, for example otoacoustic emissions tests and electronystagmography, the details of which are beyond the scope of this text.

Diseases of the ear

Diseases of the external ear

Acute otitis externa

As its name suggests otitis externa is inflammation of the external ear. It commonly follows **swimming** and is often related to pathogenic bacterial overgrowth in the canal. It may be due to eczema or psoriasis. The main symptoms are:

- Ear irritation

- Ear discharge (small, but thick, amount due to no mucus glands in external ear)

- Pain especially with pressure over tragus

- Mild conductive hearing loss

- Erythema and oedema of ear canal on examination

Treatment is with topical antibiotics and ear cleansing. Dipstick test the urine to see if the patient suffers from diabetes. Diabetics with persistent otitis externa could have **necrotising otitis externa**.

Haematoma of the pinna

This usually follows **trauma** to the ear. A haematoma (blood filled swelling) may collect between the perichondrium (membrane overlying cartilage) and cartilage. Thus it will present as a swelling of the pinna that is **fluctuant**. Normally, the perichondrium supplies the cartilage with nutrients and if it is elevated by a haematoma then the cartilage underlying it will undergo necrosis and be replaced by fibrous tissue resulting in the all famous 'cauliflower ear'.

Thus to prevent this, either a needle aspiration or incision and drainage should be undertaken. These are obviously aseptic procedures.

Diseases of the middle ear

Acute otitis media (AOM)

This is principally a disease of children aged between three and six years. It usually starts with a viral upper respiratory tract infection (URTI), thus ask about previous illnesses. The resulting nasopharyngeal oedema and inflammatory products block the Eustachian tube leading to negative middle ear pressure, and the development of a viral middle ear effusion. This effusion is unfortunately a good medium for bacteria to colonise and grow (especially Haemophilus influenza, Streptococcus pneumoniae and Moraxela catarrhalis) which then lead to suppuration (formation and discharge of pus).

To recap:

URTI → Blocked Eustachian tube → Viral effusion → 2° bacterial infection → AOM

Patients will present with:

- Otalgia
- Fever
- Malaise
- History of URTI
- Rhinitis (inflammation of nasal mucus membranes)

- Possible gastrointestinal upset (can be the only symptom)
- Conductive hearing loss (it is middle ear pathology but your average three year old is not going to complain about this)

This is an important list, try to learn it all.

Findings on examination:

- TM red
- TM bulging (absent cone of light)

Below is a picture to show what a normal eardrum looks like (Figure 1.10) and another to illustrate the appearance in a patient with acute otitis media (Figure 1.11):

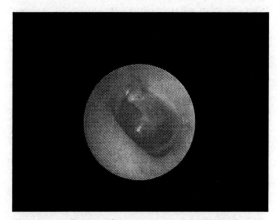

Figure 1.10 Otoscopic appearance of a normal tympanic membrane. (Reproduced with permission from Dr D Pothier)

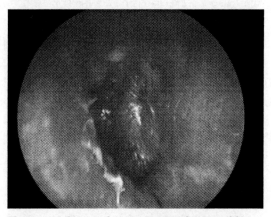

Figure 1.11 Otoscopic appearance of acute otitis media. Notice the red, bulging ear drum, with no cone of light (the others are reflections from the flash). (Reproduced with permission from Dr D Pothier)

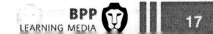

Middle and inner ear	Temporal bone	Intracranial
Tympanic membrane perforation	Acute mastoiditis	Temporal lobe abscess
Facial palsy	Gradenigo's syndrome	Cerebellar abscess
Labyrinthitis		Extradural abscess
	Subperiostial abscess	Venous sinus thrombosis
		Subdural abscess
		Meningitis

Table 1.3 The complications of AOM categorised by anatomical location

The natural history of the disease varies but resolution followed by a variable period of otitis media with effusion that can last up to three months is to be expected in the majority of cases. The eardrum will rupture in a proportion of patients leading to immediate pain relief and releasing a profuse purulent discharge. This will settle after a few days and treatment consists of fluids, analgesia and antibiotics.

If there is continuing discharge, then suspect the development of COM. Aural toilet to remove discharge, debris and obtain a clear view of the tympanic membrane is advised. Evidence of a persisting tympanic membrane perforation 12 weeks after the initial onset of ear symptoms is diagnostic of COM.

There are several important complications of AOM, and these are frequently asked about in examinations.

Acute mastoiditis occurs when the middle ear infection spreads to the mucus membranes of the mastoid bone. Infection can track through the bone often via emissary veins and come to sit between the bone surface and its periosteum leading to a subperiosteal abscess. This presents as pain behind the ear that can occasionally push the ear forward.

In the middle ear the function of the facial nerve (CN VII) may also be compromised so must be tested as described in the earlier section, *Cranial and peripheral nerve examination.* Facial paralysis if it develops usually resolves completely but it can take several months.

If the infection spreads to the inner ear then an acute suppurative labyrinthitis occurs.

Otitis media with effusion (glue ear or serous otitis media)

Before you start this let us review the Eustachian (auditory) tube (ET) as this deserves special attention with regard to middle ear disorders.

The pressures in the external ear and middle ear are both equal to atmospheric pressure, if they weren't then the TM would bulge outward or inwards resulting in pain, hearing loss and possibly perforation.

The middle ear pressure is equalised to atmospheric pressure through the Eustachian tube connecting the middle ear to the pharynx. The ending of the tube is usually shut, but during yawning, swallowing and sneezing the tube opens due to contraction of the surrounding muscle and the pressure in the middle ear equilibrates with atmospheric pressure, thus maintaining the TM in its normal position. The ET is important because it can keep the middle ear pressure constant.

In otitis media with effusion, which is a common condition and cause of hearing loss in children, ET dysfunction leads to negative pressure in the middle ear and this results in a mucosal transudate. ET dysfunction (commonly blockage) can be the result of nasopharyngeal inflammation associated with adenoiditis or nasopharyngeal obstruction secondary to neoplasm. Sticky mucus accumulates in the middle ear, splinting the eardrum and ossicles, resulting in a conductive hearing loss. The patients may not complain of any pain. The signs are:

- Dull TM
- Retracted TM – no light reflex
- Dilated blood vessels down the handle of the malleus and radially across the eardrum
- Yellow/colourless fluid behind the TM
- Hearing loss
- Bubbles behind the TM

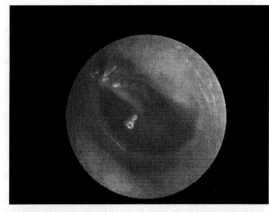

Figure 1.12 Otoscopic appearance of otitis media with effusion (OME or serous otitis media). (Reproduced with permission from Dr D Pothier.)

OME is a common sequel to acute otitis media. Decongestants, mucolytics and tonsillectomy don't help but adenoidectomy can be of benefit. The condition usually peaks between ages two and five and in 50% of children resolves over six weeks. If it doesn't resolve by three months and there is a persisting hearing loss of 25–30dB or greater in the better hearing ear then treatment consists of grommets/ventilation tubes or hearing aids.

What is a ventilation tube/grommet?

This is a small medical grade plastic tube placed into the ear drum. It is **not** is a pipe with which to drain out effusion. Its function is to equilibrate the middle ear pressure with atmospheric as it is the difference between the two that results in a middle ear effusion. In North America it is known as a pressure equalisation or ventilation tube, an 'additional Eustachian tube' because that is exactly what it is, while in the UK it is called a grommet.

It stays in place for nine to 15 months and as the TM heals it is gradually extruded. Swimming is allowed with grommets if recurrent infection is not a problem; diving is contraindicated.

Chronic otitis media (COM)

This is a very important ear disease affecting approximately 65–330 million people worldwide. It is more prevalent in the developing world but still affects 1.5%–2.6% of the population in the UK and other industrialised nations. It is divided into two types:

- Mucosal COM (COM without a cholesteatoma)
- Cholesteatoma associated COM

Patients with either type typically present with recurrent episodes of ear discharge. More than half of sufferers complain of hearing loss especially when the ear is discharging but pain is not a feature of the uncomplicated disease. The complications of COM are similar to those of AOM (see the section on AOM earlier in this chapter).

Clinical examination will usually reveal a conductive or mixed hearing loss in the affected ear. Otoscopic examination will always reveal abnormal findings though these vary with the type of COM and the activity of the disease.

Mucosal COM

These patients have a perforation in the pars tensa and may have had recurrent AOM as children. When the disease is active there will be mucopurulent discharge arising from the inflamed middle ear mucosa, as illustrated in Figure 1.13.

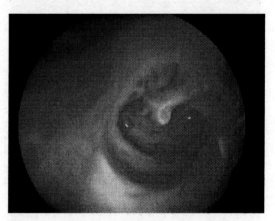

Figure 1.13 Otoscopic appearance of a subtotal tympanic membrane perforation with discharge in mucosal COM. (Reproduced with permission from Dr D Pothier.)

COM with cholesteatoma

A cholesteatoma is not as the name suggests a form of cancer. It is instead stratified squamous keratinised epithelium (skin!) growing in the middle ear and mastoid associated with infection and erosion of bone eg **ossicles (leading to hearing loss), bone over lateral semicirucular canal (leading to vertigo)**. Life-threatening

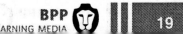

complications, meningitis, intracranial absecesses and lateral sinus thrombosis as described above for AOM can occur secondary to intracranial spread of infection. There are several hypotheses about the aetiology of cholesteatoma but these are beyond the scope of this text.

COM with cholesteatoma is characterised by the appearance of a pearly white grey mass in a defect of the pars flaccida as shown in Figure 1.14. The pars tensa in this case is also abnormal with areas of sclerosis.

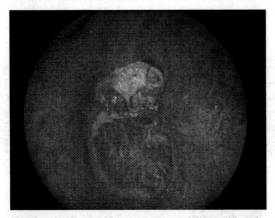

Figure 1.14 Otoscopic appearance of COM with attic cholesteatoma. (Reproduced with permission from Dr D Pothier.)

The aim of treatment is to control the recurrent episodes of ear discharge and prevent the development of complications. Topical antibiotic drops (ciprofloxacillin, an aminoquinoline) with or without steroids three times a day for a week are first line treatment. Base-line pure tone audiometery should be obtained. The majority of patients will require definitive surgical treatment with some form of tympanoplasty and mastoidectomy.

Diseases of the inner ear

Diseases of the inner ear will now be explored, and we will look at age related hearing loss (presbyacusis) and acoustic neuroma (not technically inner ear pathology) that present with sensorineural hearing loss and BPPV and vestibular neuritis that present with vertigo.

Age-related hearing loss (presbyacusis)

If we all live long enough this is something we will all get as degeneration is the proposed aetiology. It is a bilateral, progressive, symmetrical **sensorineural** hearing loss that occurs commonly after the age of 55. The pathogenesis is a gradual loss of hair cells in the cochlea and a loss of neurones in the cochlear nerve. More high frequency hearing is lost than low frequency hearing. This makes speech comprehension very difficult (especially consonants), and difficulty in distinguishing speech is an early symptom especially in background noise.

Hearing aids are the mainstay of treatment. Remember, the hearing loss is bilateral; if you find a unilateral hearing loss think instead of an acoustic neuroma.

Acoustic neuroma (vestibular schwannoma)

This is a benign tumour of Schwann cells arising from the vestibular division of the vestibulocochlear (VIII) nerve. The lesion is situated in the internal auditory canal (meatus) or the angle between the cerebellum and pons – cerebellopontine angle.

The most common presenting symptoms are unilateral sensorineural hearing loss and tinnitus. These are directly related to involvement of CN VIII. In far advanced disease, rarely encountered nowadays patients may have

- Paraesthesia secondary to pressure on CN V

- Ataxia, nystagmus related to cerebellar compression

- Headache from raised intracranial pressure (a killer), due to obstruction of CSF flow through the aqueduct/4th ventricle

An MRI head scan to investigate the internal auditory meatus is the definitive investigation. Treatment options are active monitoring with serial MRI scans (not all lesions are growing), surgical removal or stereotactic radiosurgery (radiation treatment).

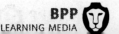

Benign Paroxysmal Positional Vertigo (BPPV)

This is one of the commonest causes of vertigo (see section on vertigo). Patients present at any age with a history of episodic vertigo (lasting seconds to a minute) precipitated by changes in head position. There may be a history of a preceding minor head injury. They report vertigo being triggered by changing position in bed, looking up or down. In many cases the attacks will settle spontaneously with time. When the condition persists, you will be able to elicit a positive response on Dix-Hallpike testing (see the section on the Dix-Hallpike test).

One theory attributes the condition to otolith (calcium) particles from the cupola of the semicircular canal that have broken free and come to lie within the canal. As the patient changes their head position these particles collide with the cupola distorting the sensory hair cells more than usual and precipitating vertigo. First line treatment is with particle repositioning manoeuvres, such as the Epeley, that move the offending particles into the vestibule proper away from the semicircular canal sensory epithelium. Surgery (semicircular canal compression) is reserved for resistant cases and compresses the membranous semicircular canal to prevent any further particle movement along it, after removing the overlying bony cover.

Vestibular neuritis

This alarming condition presents with the sudden onset of incapacitating vertigo, nausea and vomiting classically following an upper respiratory tract infection. There may be a history of similar symptoms in personal contacts as it is thought to be viral in origin. Hearing is unaffected. The vertigo persists for 48 to 72 hours and any movement makes the symptoms worse. Patients therefore usually confine themselves to bed. Gaze nystagmus may be elicited if the patient is seen in the acute phase. The vertigo gradually settles over two to four days and the patient is able to get out of bed but remains very unsteady for a week or more.

Evidence of unilateral vestibular weakness can be elicited on Head thrust, Rhomberg's and/or the stepping gait clinical tests. Treatment in the acute phase consists of vestibular sedatives such as prochlorperazine. This should not be continued long term once the nausea and vomiting has settled as treatment should then be directed to promoting compensation by increasing the sensitivity of any residual vestibular function in the contra-lateral ear, input from muscle and joint proprioceptors, vision and the integration of the altered pattern of balance sensory input on higher balance centres in the brain. Vestibular rehabilitation exercises hasten compensation.

Neoplasms of the ear and temporal bone

These are rare. Presenting features are a chronic discharging ear resisitant to treatment and pain in patients 50 years of age and older. Patients present late and diagnosis is delayed because the common presenting feature of a discharging ear is more usually diagnosed as otitis externa. Biospsy of any suspicious masses arising from the ear canal including aural polyps in a chronically discharging ear is the key to obtaining the histological diagnosis. Squamous cell carcinoma is the predominant histological type. Clinical examination should look for spread or origin in the parotid gland and cervical lymphadenopathy. Check for facial nerve and lower cranial nerve involvement. Investigations are aimed at determining local extent and metastic spread thus CT and MRI imaging of the temporal bone and head are undertaken in addition to a metastic screen. Treatment is temporal bone resection and radiotherapy but the five-year survival is less than 50% in large series.

Red flags in otology

The patient requires an urgent referral to an Otolaryngologist if he or she has one of the following symptoms or signs:

- Unilateral persistant ear discharge especially if painful (cancer of the temporal bone)

- Sudden unilateral sensorineural hearing loss (a proportion of cases can be treated with intratympanic or systemic steroids)

- Mastoiditis, facial palsy or features suggestive of complicated acute or COM (patient at greater risk of developing a fatal intracranial complication and requires consideration for surgical treatment)

What to do in an OSCE

You could be asked to take a history from a patient with a primary complaint related to the ears or hearing and/or undertake a clinical examination of the patient's ears and hearing. An ear history will require you to ask the main questions in the *Clinical history* section and, with a rough idea of the basic pathologies, you should be fine.

Ensure that you familiarise yourself with your medical school or local hospital's policy on dress for clinical medical students as these vary and are likely to be enforced in a clinical examination. In North America for example a clean white laboratory coat may be expected but in the UK no coats of any type should be worn and the upper limbs below the elbows should be bare (no watches, but wedding rings are allowed). Remember to bring your Student Doctor ID badge and the necessary equipment (eg pen and pen torch). Don't panic, it won't help, just stay focused on the following and all will be fine:

- Inspection
- Otoscope
- Basic hearing tests
- Rinne, Weber
- Cranial nerves

Scenario

In a typical scenario you may be asked to examine a patient's ears.

You should adopt an ordered approach to avoid missing elements of the clinical examinition. Wash your hands, **introduce yourself** and ask the patient for **permission** to examine him/her.

Ask if they are in **any pain** at the start, this is very important. If they say 'yes', tell them you'll try to be gentle and apologise in advance for hurting them just in case, eg 'Okay [name], I'll try to be as gentle as I can, but if I do hurt you I don't mean to and please let me know and I'll stop'.

Following the formalities, start off with **inspection** and tell the examiner what you are doing (refer to the section on *Clinical examination*).

Then move onto the **otoscope**. Choose and fit an appropriate end-piece and check the power. Let the patient know what you are doing and let them know that it may be uncomfortable (most of the marks in an OSCE depend on your manner with the patient). Then pull the pinna up and back and have a look. Say what you can see, even if it is nothing, but **don't lie!** For example, if you say that wax is obstructing your view the examiners will know whether this is the case as they have probably already looked at the patient. Try to describe the TM, say what you can see eg cone of light, pars tensa etc. Remember to examine both ears.

Do the clinical tests of hearing followed by the **Rinne** and **Weber** tuning fork tests. Ask for a 512Hz or 256Hz tuning fork if you haven't got one available. If you have time, check **facial nerve** function.

Finish off by thanking the patient. Be prepared to describe your findings in a succinct and ordered fashion. While undertaking the examination you should be thinking of a potential diagnosis and ideally a differential. It should be clear from the instructions at the start of the station if you will be required to summarise your findings including potential diagnoses. In a clinical examination arriving at the correct diagnosis after a properly conducted examination and precise summary of one's findings is likely to result in a perfect score.

References

Acuin, J. World Health Organisation (WHO) (2004) *Chronic Suppurative Otitis Media – Burden of Illness and Management Options.* [Online] WHO. Available at: www.who.int/pbd/deafness/activities/hearing_care/otitis_media.pdf [Accessed 17 April 2012].

Bibas AG, Ward V and Gleeson MJ. Squamous cell carcinoma of the temporal bone. *J Laryngol Otol* 2008; Nov 122(11): 1156–6. Available online at: www.ncbi.nlm.nih.gov/pubmed/18177533 [Accessed 17 April 2012].

Browning GG and Gatehouse S. The prevalence of middle ear disease in the adult British population. *Clin Otolaryngol* 1992; 17(4): 317–21.

Lempert T, Gresty MA and Bronstein AM. Benign positional vertigo: recognition and treatment. *BMJ* 1995 Aug 19; 311(7003): 489–91.

McDonald S, Langton Hewer CD and Nunez DA. Grommets (ventilation tubes) for recurrent acute otitis media in children. *Cochrane Database Syst Rev* 2008 Oct 8; (4): CD004741. Review. Available online at: www.ncbi.nlm.nih.gov/pubmed/18843668 [Accessed 17 April 2012].

National Institute for Health and Clinical Excellence (guideline 60) (Feb 2008) *Surgical Management of Otitis Media with Effusion in Children.* [Online] NICE. Available at: www.nice.org.uk/nicemedia/live/11928/39564/39564.pdf [Accessed 30 August 2011].

Subcommittee on Management of Acute Otitis Media. Diagnosis and management of acute otitis media. *American Academy of Pediatrics. Pediatrics* 2004; 113(5): 1451–65. Available online at: http://pediatrics.aappublications.org/content/113/5/1451.full [Accessed 17 April 2012].

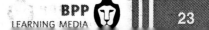

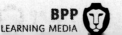

Chapter 2

Nose – rhinology

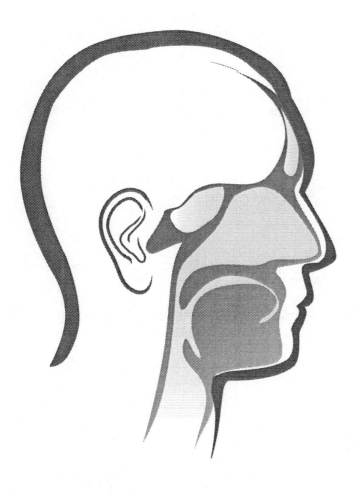

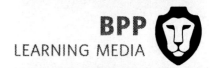

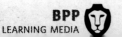

Introduction

The nose is the organ of olfaction (smell) and respiration. It also adds resonance to the voice (which is why your voice changes when you have a cold/blocked nose) and is the site of drainage of the paranasal sinuses and tear ducts (into the lateral nasal wall).

Don't forget respiration, as everyone's first instinct is to answer that smell is the only function of the nose. Olfaction is of more importance to animals lower in the phylogenetic (evolutionary) scale than humans and is one of the first senses to arise. Its importance in determining behaviour is apparent from connections of the olfactory nerve (Cranial Nerve I) to the limbic system (amygdala specifically).

Anatomy and physiology of the nose and smell

The nose consists of an external framework enclosing a partitioned internal cavity. The median nasal septum running from the nostrils (nares) to the back of the throat separates the right and left nasal cavities. The upper part of the supporting nasal framework consists of the paired nasal bones and the lower part of cartilages. The paired alar cartilages surrounding the nares contribute to the definition of the nasal tip. The upper lateral nasal cartilages sit between the alar cartilages and the nasal bones.

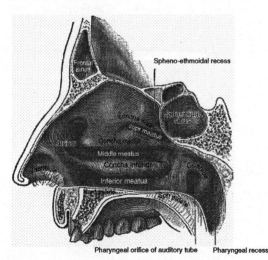

Figure 2.1 The lateral nasal wall
Gray H (1918) Anatomy of the Human Body, 20th edition, Lea & Febiger, Philadelphia
(This image is in the public domain because its copyright had expired. This applies worldwide.)

The nares entrance (vestibule) is lined by normal hair bearing skin (vibrissae). The vibrissae help to prevent the entry of large particulate matter into the nose. Respiratory epithelium lines the nasal cavity deep to the vestibule. While the septum is generally a smooth surface except where deflections (deviations) occur, the lateral nasal wall consists of a number of projections and hollows.

Three bones termed conchae (singular concha) or turbinates project medially into the nasal cavity from each lateral nasal wall. The turbinates, like the rest of nasal cavity beyond the vestibule, are covered by normal respiratory mucosa and increase the surface area available for heat and moisture exchange in the nose.

The nose has a rich blood supply. The main artery of the nasal cavity is the **sphenopalatine** branch of the maxillary artery (which enters through the maxillary foramen). It anastomoses with the following arteries:

- Palatine artery
- Ethmoidal arteries – anterior and posterior
- Labial artery

(Mnemonic: SPEL)

This anastomosis forms what is called Kiesselbach's plexus, located on the lower anterior part of the septum – the famous **Little's area** – a common site for nosebleeds (epistaxis; refer to the section on *Diseases of the nose and sinuses* later in this chapter).

The large surface area and rich blood supply serve to warm, clean and moisten the air that comes into the nose. Particulate matter is trapped by the cilia that project from cells in the mucus membrane. The cilia, as their counterparts in the lung, sway back and forth thus projecting the dirt backward to the pharynx to be swallowed (and destroyed by gastric acid). This is a valuable defence mechanism designed to prevent respiratory infections. The nasal equivalent to the respiratory cough reflex is sneezing. This ejects the contents of the nasal cavity to the outside world. It does this in response to irritation (for example a strong eau de toilette/ aftershave).

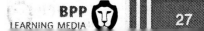

How do we smell?

Olfactory receptors are specialised cilia containing nerve cells which lie in the olfactory epithelium of the nasal cavity. These have axons which assemble into several fascicles which enter the skull on the perforated cribriform plate of the ethmoid bone. From here they attach to the olfactory bulb on the inferior surface of the frontal lobe. Thus a fracture of the cribriform plate may lead to anosmia (loss of the sense of smell). Although this may seem trivial, it isn't. One reason is that you will lose the flavour of foods. The constituents eg sweet and salt, are fine (CN VII) but you will lose the majority of the major flavour cues and hence one of life's pleasures. More important is the health and safety impairment suffered by the anosmic patient. In the USA and UK domestic and small industry gas supplies are treated with an odourant to allow users to detect leakage. Anosmic patients are unable to identify this smell, putting their employment at risk in some instances, in addition to their safety in the home.

What is special about olfactory receptor cells is that they are the only neurones in adult humans which undergo continuous neurogenesis ie they are continuously replaced. The olfactory pathways terminate in the primary olfactory cortex of the uncus in the temporal lobe and in the amygdala.

What is smell? Smell is a sensory perception of odours (chemicals). Initially the odourant molecules enter the nasal cavity and dissolve in the mucus. They then bind to receptors present on the olfactory cilia. The receptors are specific for particular odourant molecules. Following this binding, an intracellular cascade takes place involving guanine diphosphate (GDP) and so forth, resulting in the opening of a sodium channel and the cell depolarising (ENa^+ approximately +40mV). The resulting action potentials generated from the binding of the odour to the receptor, are transmitted from the olfactory sensors to the bulb. There, interneurones integrate the information from sensors and pass the signal to higher central pathways involving the lateral olfactory stria and terminating in the relevant areas of cortex (as for the ear and everything else for that matter, the brain 'smells' not the nose – smell is a sensory perception).

The receptors for smell are high up in the nose which is why when you sniff you can smell better than just gently breathing the odour in.

Sinuses

Sinuses are hollow chambers that have foramina for draining into the nose. Their function is still controversial, perhaps they make the skull lighter, aid in phonation or act as shock absorbers to redistribute the forces of blunt trauma away from the orbit and so protect the eye. There are four groups of sinuses and you really ought to know them all. They are:

- Frontal
- Ethmoid
- Maxillary
- Sphenoid

They are lined by respiratory epithelium. Unfortunately the genetic design plan is better than the end product because the drainage arrangement is prone to getting blocked, resulting in infection and inflammation. The maxillary sinus drains into the middle meatus of the nasal cavity (space below the middle concha). It drains through a hole (an ostium), which is at the superior part of the sinus. Drainage through the ostium is therefore not by gravity as the opening is too high up but rather by active directional beating of the cilia towards the ostium. Thus maxillary sinus drainage is dependent on normal ciliary function, one of the first casualties of infection. Evidence and practice suggests that far less good comes of the sinuses than bad.

Clinical history

The main areas to probe in a nasal history are shown below; each will be discussed in more detail.

- Airway obstruction
- Runny nose (rhinorrhoea) – mucus/blood
- Loss of smell
- Facial pain
- Sneezing
- Snoring

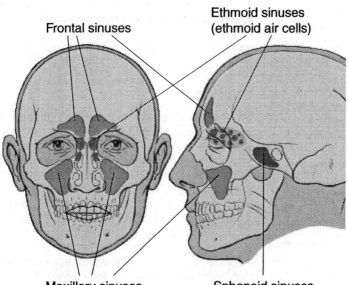

Frontal sinuses

Ethmoid sinuses
(ethmoid air cells)

Maxillary sinuses

Sphenoid sinuses

Figure 2.2: The location of the sinuses

As part of the full history you should also ask about:

- The variability of symptoms – seasonal versus perennial (all year)

- The pattern of nasal obstruction

- Previous surgery

- Trauma

- Drug history

- Allergies/atopic diseases (asthma, eczema)

- Pets at home

- Occupation

- Smoking history

- General medical conditions eg diabetes, acromegaly, hypothyroidism

- Effect of nasal symptoms on eating, speech and sleep

Airways obstruction

This is an important and distressing symptom, especially in children as they are obligate nasal breathers. You ought to ask clarifiying questions to determine:

- Site
- Onset
- Character
- Alleviating factors
- Exacerbating factors
- Timing
- Severity
- Associated factors

Associated symptoms include rhinorrhoea, post-nasal drip, sneezing, itching and facial pain.

Rhinorrhoea

Again, use the clarifying questions (outlined in the subsection on *Airways obstruction* above). Find out if the discharge is mucus or blood. The presence of a thick, coloured nasal discharge is indicative of infective rhinosinusitis. Is there clear fluid? This could be CSF. If it is, the descriptive term is CSF rhinorrhoea and may be post-traumatic due to a fracture of the cribriform plate tearing part of the meninges or spontaneous (related to a congenital skull base defect or benign intracranial hypertension).

Anosmia

Start with the same clarifying questions as described under the section on *Airways obstruction* above. Ask about associated symptoms specifically nasal blockage and rhinorrhoea. Conditions leading to an olfactory conduction block, due to the failure of odourant molecules getting to the olfactory sensitive epithelium, account for the majority of cases of hyposmia (reduced smell sensitivity) or anosmia. Upper respiratory tract infections (the common cold), allergic and non-allergic rhinitis and nasal polyps are examples.

Patients with neurosensory olfactory dysfunction present much less commonly. In this group acquired causes trauma, tumour and degenerative disorders along with congenital causes should be considered. Therefore ask about head trauma that can lead to damage to the olfactory nerves or bulb. Enquire about other cranial nerve symptoms such as visual disturbance and headache. Loss of smell is a frequent symptom in Alzheimer's and Parkinson's diseases, it predates the onset of the motor features in the latter condition. A family history of anosmia may help identify rare causes for anosmia such as hypogonadotrophic hypogonadism.

Facial pain

This is important, and you must take a detailed history not only of the pain but of associated symptoms as well such as sneezing, pruritus (itching) and rhinorrhoea. Ask what makes the pain better and when it comes on. Is it related to the seasons? Are there any other neurological symptoms such as an aura (implying migraine)? Try to assess the patietnt's mood, as facial pain may be related to depression. The facial pain associated with sinusitis is usually in the form of a dull ache/sense of pressure, which gets worse with a cold and on bending forward/stooping. It is also associated with other symptoms of sinusitis such as a coloured, thick nasal discharge and nasal obstruction.

Sneezing

Sneezing is seldom an isolated symptom so ask about other nasal symptoms (nasal obstruction, rhinorrhoea, facial pain etc) to arrive at a possible cause.

Snoring

This is an important and distressing symptom that many patients find disturbing and not funny, so be sympathetic. A history from a partner may help. Snoring may be caused by obstructive sleep apnoea (OSA). This is an upper airways disease (obstruction) that occurs during sleep. The reason being, that the pharyngeal and laryngeal muscles normally maintain the patency of the upper airway during inspiration. During sleep the muscle tone is reduced and the upper airways may be sucked in, resulting in the sound and poor quality of sleep that leaves the patient very tired during the day. It may be caused by enlargement of the tongue as occurs in acromegaly, hypothyroidism and Trisomy 21 (Down's syndrome).

Ask about a recent increase in the patient's weight/body mass index, a history of disturbed sleep and excessive day time tiredness/somnolence. OSA is associated with hypertension, and alcohol and cigarette consumption. So do ask about these also. Ask how it has affected the patient's personal life to get an idea of how big the problem is. Rarely, nocturia may be a feature.

Clinical examination

You should be able to examine the nose in an OSCE. It is also especially important in A&E or if you do an ENT rotation and of course in general practice.

The rules that apply to any other system examination are modified:

Inspection, palpation, and functional assessment should be undertaken but inspection is most important.

Most of the nose exam is inspection. First inspect with your eyes alone, then with a wide ended speculum attached to the otoscope or a Thudicum speculum (a speculum used to retract the alar cartilage) and a separate light source. Finally, assess airflow obstruction by, for example, using a cold metal tongue depressor. Don't forget to introduce yourself and to obtain the patient's permission to undertake the examination. Ask if the nose is painful or tender to touch.

Inspection

First look at the nose and face from a distance and ask the patient to remove their spectacles. Look at the profile as well as the front and look for:

- Deviations and deformities
- Growths
- Scars
- Redness
- Discharge (colour, smell)

To inspect the front of the nose, lift the tip with the thumb of your left hand while resting the tips of the fingers on the patient's forehead and look inside (this may reveal a severe deflection of the nasal septum or an intranasal mass presenting in the vestibule). Inspection will be aided by using a bright light either held in your right hand or carried on a headband.

A further view into the nose (anterior rhinoscopy) can be obtained most safely for the non-otolaryngologist by gently introducing the tip of a wide ended aural speculum attached to the otoscope into the nostril while holding the nasal tip up. You can use the Thudicum speculum to retract the alar cartilage and obtain a better view; however we recommend that you ask an otolaryngologist to demonstrate its use and that you practise using the instrument under supervision before trying to use it on your own. Inappropriate use will cause the patient discomfort!

While inspecting or undertaking anterior rhinoscopy you should see the nasal septum in the midline and the turbinates on the lateral nasal wall. Look for evidence of inflammation and if the septum is straight or not, ie is there a septal deviation? Are there any foreign bodies? You ought to be able to see the inferior turbinate (pink/mucosal in colour), but are less likely to see the middle one.

Palpation

If there is an apparent deviation of the external nasal structure, gentle palpation over the nasal skeleton can help to determine if it is due to a bony or cartilaginous deformity. Palpation with a probe such as the working end of a Jobson-Horne probe can be used to distinguish the turbinates from nasal polyps or determine if nasal polyps or other nasal masses arise from the nasal septum or lateral nasal wall. The turbinates are exquisitely sensitive to touch via a speculum (or anything else for that matter) unlike for example a polyp which is insensate and usually grey/yellow in colour.

Functional assessment

Finish the examination by assessing nasal airflow. One method that is easy to master is to take a cold metal tongue depressor and place it on the patient's philtrum (midline grove in the upper lip) directly under the nose and ask the patient to breathe normally through the nose. If there is normal air flow and no obstruction then both nostrils should make the tongue depressor cloudy in two reciprocal circles. However, if one nostril is completely blocked then only one foggy circle will appear on the tongue depressor, related to the non-obstructed nostril.

You wouldn't assess smell in a routine clinical examination of the nose although it is undertaken in specialist clinics.

Do practise the above as you will get better the more times you undertake a full nasal clinical assessment.

Diseases of the nose and sinuses

The main pathologies explored here are allergic rhinitis, vasomotor rhinitis, epistaxis, nasal polyps, acute sinusitis, chronic rhino-sinusitis and neoplasms of the nose.

Allergic rhinitis

This is one disease where there is a lot of literature, so the main clinical features will be addressed, but not the basic science concerning antibodies etc.

Allergic rhinitis may be classified into seasonal and perennial. Symptoms are usually bilateral and variable in severity. In cases of grass and tree pollen allergy, symptoms are proportional to the levels of pollen in the environment. Patients often have other features of atopy such as eczema or asthma. A young age of onset (before 20 years of age) and family history of allergy is common. The symptoms are:

- Rhinorrhoea
- Sneezing
- Pruritus of nose, eyes or throat
- Nasal congestion
- Eye tearing

The signs would be:

- Pale blue, boggy mucosa
- Colourless discharge
- Swollen turbinates
- Allergic salute (the tilting up of the nasal tip by the base of the hand)
- Allergic dorsal skin crease

Skin prick allergen challenge tests or blood tests for specific antibodies can be used to identify the allergen/s. Allergen avoidance, intra-nasal steroids and systemic anti-histamines are the usual treatment. The accumulating evidence of the effectiveness and safety of sublingual immunotherapy at least in adults increases the acceptability and likelihood that desensitisation will be increasingly used in these patients.

Vasomotor rhinitis

This is a type of non-allergic rhinitis. It is characterised by the presence of rhinitis but without an obvious cause such as allergy, infection or underlying structural nasal abnormality. It is perennial, more common in women and in patients older than 20 years. It is thought to be related to changes in autonomic tone of the arteriolar capillary muscle. Normally, the sympathetic nervous system (SNS) causes vasoconstriction and parasympathetic (PSNS) the opposite. What happens in this pathology is that there is either a fall in the SNS tone or increase in the PSNS tone, which causes vasodilatation and hence an increase in capillary hydrostatic pressure resulting in a profuse, watery nasal secretion usually manifest as post-nasal drip.

The symptoms are triggered by exposure to respiratory irritants such as cigarette smoke and strong perfumes but also changes in temperature and atmospheric pressure.

There are other forms of non-allergic rhinitis caused by drugs and hormones (eg rhinitis of pregnancy) to be considered amongst the differential diagnoses.

The symptoms are:

- Variable bilateral obstruction
- Post nasal drip
- Exacerbated by tobacco, perfume and temperature change (distinguishes from allergic rhinitis)
- Not much itching (distinguishes from allergic rhinitis)

The signs of vasomotor rhinitis are:

- Congestion of nasal mucosa
- No other abnormality detected

Epistaxis (nosebleed)

Epistaxis can be an emergency and, as with all emergencies, the golden rule is **ABC** – airway, breathing and circulation.

The aetiology could be:

- Trauma including forceful blowing of nose
- Nose picking
- Nasal vestibulitis
- Rhinitis
- NSAIDs or aspirin
- Nasal foreign body
- Coagulopathy
- Nasal surgery
- Neoplasia
- Cocaine abuse
- Hypertension (controversial)

Bleeding in children especially if recurrent is usually from Little's area (refer to the *Anatomy and physiology* section). In such cases the key is to put pressure on the area by squeezing the cartilaginous (inferior) part of the nose from both sides between the thumb and forefinger. Advise the patient to lean the head forward (not backward – to prevent aspiration of blood).

Decongestion of the nasal mucosa with topical vasoconstrictors aids detailed examination to identify a bleeding point, that can then be cauterised with silver nitrate. If a discrete bleeding point cannot be identified, pack the nose with the nasal packs (there are several different types)

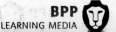

available in your hospital. Don't forget ABC in the patient presenting with an acute epistaxis: that's the life saver.

In the older patient and after nasal bone injury, bleeds are usually from further back in the nose and so pressure on Little's area isn't helpful. Rather, ice on the nose as a first aid should be followed by examination to identify a vessel to be cauterised, and if this fails, nasal packing. Advise the patient to breathe through the mouth, supplemental oxygen delivered by a face mask may be required as nasal packing is associated with hypoxia especially in older patients.

If bleeding is not controlled, arterial ligation in theatre, either sphenopalatine under endoscopic control and/or anterior ethmoid, is the next step.

Nasal polyps

These are fluid filled sacs from the prolapsed lining of the ethmoid sinuses. They are soft lobulated masses (not neoplasm) that lead to nasal obstruction. They are more common in the over 40s. In some patients the nasal polyps are one element in a triad, termed Samter's Triad which is the combination of aspirin allergy, nasal polyps and asthma. Thus do ask about asthma and aspirin allergy in the history. Chronic Rhinosinusitis (CRS) is associated either as a causative factor or a consequence due to obstruction of sinus outlet drainage. The finding of nasal polyps on examination clinches the diagnosis.

The symptoms are:

- Nasal blockage
- Watery rhinorrhoea
- Post-nasal drip
- Sneezing
- Headache
- Change in voice
- Loss of smell
- Taste disturbance

The signs of nasal polyps are:

- Widening external nostrils if large
- Painless, mobile, soft, lobulated mass.
- Usually bilateral
- Commonly arises from the middle meatus

Note. If there is a unilateral polyp with an irregular appearance and (especially) if it is bleeding/ulcerating, malignancy **must** be ruled out.

Medical treatment consists of antibiotics, topical and systemic steroids. Surgery to remove the polyps, either endoscopic polypectomy alone or with more extensive nasal sinus surgery, is often required. Unfortunately they commonly recur and therefore patients are prescribed long-term topical steroid therapy to stabilise the nasal lining and extend the length of time to recurrence.

Acute sinusitis

This is a secondary bacterial infection following a viral infection. The duration of symptoms is more than ten days but less than 12 weeks. It is acute inflammation of the sinuses but involves the lining of the nose as well (rhinosinusitis). Normally, the cilia sweep mucus from the sinuses into the nose. If however a viral infection (eg influenza, rhinovirus) depresses ciliary activity, and the associated oedema narrows the ostium, this results in an accumulation of mucus in the sinus. The static mucus is a good culture medium for bacteria and a secondary infection may take over which depresses cilia function further. Alternative routes of infection include bacterial spread from an infected molar tooth root in the floor of the maxillary sinus, and forceful entry of dirty water into the frontal sinus from jumping foot first into the water. Other predisposing risk factors for acute sinusitis, which you can tease out are:

- Polyps
- Septal deviation
- Immunosuppression
- Cystic fibrosis
- Samter's Triad
- Allergic rhinitis

Try to remember about three of these, as they are important.

The symptoms of Acute Rhinosinusitis (ARS) are:

- Yellow/green coloured rhinorrhoea
- Fever, fatigue
- Sinus tenderness
- Nasal obstruction
- Anosmia
- Mouth breathing
- Aching pain

The signs are:

- Inflammation of nasal mucosa (enlarged turbinates)
- Nasal discharge
- Percussion tenderness of sinus

Treatment consists of analgesia, steroids, topical decongestants but not oral antihistamines. If there is evidence of a bacterial infection (usually lasts longer, >10 days as opposed to self-limiting viral infections) antibiotics may be indicated. Surgery is not usually indicated for acute sinusitis.

Chronic Rhinosinusitis (CRS)

The primary symptoms are:

- Rhinorrhea
- Nasal obstruction
- Facial pain
- Post nasal drip (catarrh)
- Anosmia

Associated symptoms include

- Chronic cough
- Halitosis
- Hoarse voice
- Hearing loss

The signs are:

- Nasal mucosal inflammation
- Purulent nasal discharge especially arising from the middle meatus

CRS is defined by the persistence of the above symptoms and signs beyond three months. The aetiology is multifactorial but there is invariably associated bacterial or fungal infection. Predisposing conditions include mucosal inflammation secondary to allergic rhinitis; ciliary dysfunction eg cystic fibrosis; anatomical anomalies eg nasal septal deviation, and host factors such as smoking.

First line treatment includes the use of a topical steroid spray for a period of 12 weeks. In the presence of a purulent nasal discharge, primary care physicians should also prescribe patients a four-week course of a broad spectrum antibiotic. Patients who fail such treatment should be reviewed by an otolaryngologist who would perform a nasal endoscopy and may prescribe a longer course of antibiotics eg macrolides such as clarithromycin

(up to a total of 12 weeks). Symptom control can also be improved with analgesics, nasal saline douching and allergen avoidance in the allergic patient. Patients who fail to respond to medical management should be considered for surgical treatment in the form of functional endoscopic sinus surgery (FESS).

FESS is undertaken to promote sinus drainage and aeration by unblocking and widening the natural sinus ostia. The risks of sinus surgery in trained hands are low but patients should be warned of the risks of bleeding, facial bruising, and visual disturbance: either double vision (diplopia) or loss of vision and brain injury.

Causes of a runny nose (rhinorrhoea)

You should know a few causes by now (hopefully). A good rhinological history will help identify many causes. Important causes of a runny nose are as follows:

- Bacterial/viral infection of upper respiratory tract
- Allergic rhinitis
- Non-allergic rhinitis (including vasomotor rhinitis)
- Acute sinusitis
- Chronic Rhinosinusitis
- Nasal polyps
- Foreign body (unilateral rhinorrhoea)
- Rhinitis medicamentosa (due to too many decongestants that work via vasoconstriction)
- Nasal tumour (blood-stained rhinorrhoea)
- Trauma (CSF rhinorrhoea)
- Cystic fibrosis
- Drugs

Neoplasms of the nose and sinuses

Tumours of the nose and sinuses are rare. These could be benign or malignant. Cancer of the nose and sinuses is exceedingly rare and comprises

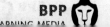

only about 5% of head and neck cancers. Beware of patients presenting with unilateral nasal or sinus symptoms as this could be caused by an underlying sino-nasal tumour.

Red flags in rhinology

The patient requires an urgent referral to an otolaryngologist if he or she has one of the following symptoms or signs:

- Unilateral nasal obstruction with purulent nasal discharge which may or may not be blood stained
- Unilateral nasal mass or polyp
- Unilateral facial swelling
- Proptosis/unilateral visual symptoms
- Ill-fitting dentures of recent onset

What to do in an OSCE

The rhinology OSCE question at the medical student level is more likely to require you to take a history from a patient with nasal symptoms rather than undertake a nasal examination. If you are required to take a history, then start first by introducing yourself to the patient and obtaining their verbal consent to a clinical interview. This is an appropriate time to ascertain their age and

occupation, both of which may provide diagnostic clues, for example a head gardener presenting with rhinorrhoea. Make contempraneous notes as you elicit the history not only as an aide memoire to your findings, but to also allow you hopefully to spot the questions you have forgotten to ask.

Ask the patient (or actor as it is common for medical schools to engage professional actors for this type of station to improve the consistency of the responses to the medical students' questions) to describe their main problem in their own words – this will allow you to identify the main presenting complaint. You need to clarify this further in terms of speed of onset, duration, variability, severity, exacerbating, relieving and associated factors etc (refer to the section on *Airways obstruction*). The novice often neglects to ask about associated factors, medication used, asthma or other features of atopy although these make a significant contribution to determining the likely diagnosis.

Remember the point of taking a clinical history is to obtain a diagnosis, therefore you are looking for both important positive and negative responses to help pinpoint the diagnosis. Be prepared to give the examiner a succinct synopsis of your findings (as if you were presenting the case on a ward round or in the clinic to one of your seniors). Knowledge of at least the features of the diseases discussed in the section *Diseases of the nose and sinuses* is essential to perform well at this station.

References

Fokkens W, et al EAACI position paper on rhinosinusitis and nasal polyps executive summary. *Allergy* 2005; 60(5): 583–601.

Khalil, HS, Nunez, DA. Functional endoscopic sinus surgery for Chronic Rhinosinusitis. *Cochrane Database Syst Rev.* 2006; 3: 1–18

Lopatin AS, Kapitanov DN and Potapov AA. Endonasal endoscopic repair of spontaneous cerebrospinal fluid leaks. *Arch Otolaryngol Head Neck Surg.* 2003;129: 859–863

Munro JF and Campbell IW (2000) *Macleod's Clinical Examination.* Churchill Livingstone.

Report of the Rhinosinusitis Task Force Committee meeting. Alexandria, Virginia, August 17, 1996. *Otolaryngol Head Neck Surg.* 1997 Sep; 117(3 Pt 2): S1–68.

Settipane RA. Rhinitis: a dose of epidemiological reality. *Allergy Asthma Proc.* 2003 May–Jun; 24(3): 147–54.

Thomas M, et al on behalf of the European position paper on rhinosinusitis and nasal polyps group. EPOS primary care guidelines: European position paper on the primary care diagnosis and management of rhinosinusitis and nasal polyps 2007 – a summary. *Prim Care Respir J.* 2008 Jun; 17(2): 79–89.

Wattendorf E, et al Olfactory impairment predicts brain atrophy in Parkinson's disease. *J Neurosci.* (Dec 2009) 9; 29(49): 15410–3.

Wilson DR, Torres LI and Durham SR. Sublingual immunotherapy for allergic rhinitis. *Cochrane Database Syst Rev.* 2003; (2): CD002893.

Chapter 3

Throat – laryngology

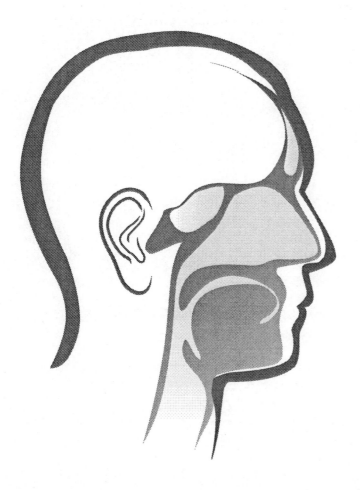

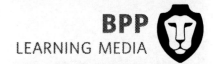

Introduction

When we talk about the throat we are really talking about the pharynx. In this chapter, we will explore the basic science and then move on to look at the clinical evaluation of both the pharynx and larynx. This is followed by a discussion of the pathology of both structures after which we then look at the neck.

Throat

Anatomy and physiology of the pharynx

The pharynx is the cavity at the back of the nose, mouth and larynx. It consists of a $7\frac{1}{2}$ cm long fibromuscular tube that extends from the base of the skull (see Figure 3.1) to the inferior border of the cricoid cartilage at the level of C6. It opens into the oesophagus at its inferior end.

The part of the pharynx that lies at the back of the nose, ie above the level of the palate is the nasopharynx. The part of the pharynx beyond the mouth (commonly referred to as the throat when examined through the mouth, hence throat swabs) is the oropharynx. The hypopharynx is below the oropharynx, lying behind the larynx and is the last part of the pharynx before the start of the oesophagus.

The pharynx is lined with a mucus membrane that is respiratory (pseudostratified columnar) in the nasopharynx, but changes to non-keratinising stratified squamous epithelium in the parts that are exposed to food (the oro and hypopharynx). To remind you of the regional anatomy see Figure 3.1.

It looks long and complex but you will already know most of the structures. Let us briefly talk about the anatomy and physiology of the pharynx and the larynx, as these are important structures to understand. Once you understand their normal function, pathology becomes a lot easier to follow.

Muscles of the pharynx

The muscle layers of the pharynx are formed by the:

*   Outer circular pharyngeal constrictor muscle layer

*   Inner longitudinal muscle layer

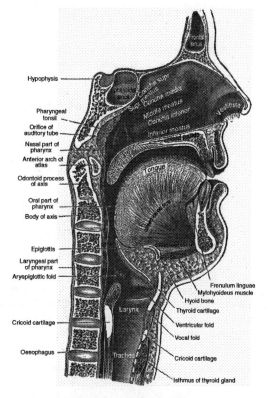

Figure 3.1 Saggital view of the pharynx Gray H (1918) Anatomy of the Human Body, 20th edition, Lea & Febiger, Philadelphia *(This image is in the public domain because its copyright had expired. This applies worldwide)*

There are three constrictor muscles named simply the superior, middle and inferior constrictors and their main function is to propel the food bolus downwards (this part of the swallowing reflex is under initial **voluntary** control and the muscle is striated).

There are likewise three longitudinal albeit paired muscles, salpingopharyngeus, stylopharyngeus and palatopharyngeus (tip: just add -pharyngeus to salpingo, stylo and palato). Most of these muscles elevate the pharynx during swallowing.

Remember, what takes place in swallowing (or what your body does to direct the passage of the food bolus):

- Protect the nasal airway from food through the action of the soft palate.
- Protect the lower airway via laryngeal mechanisms that include contraction of the laryngeal inlet and elevation of the larynx so bringing the epiglottis to lie like a lid over the inlet.
- Relax the upper oesophageal sphincter to allow the food to proceed into the digestive tract proper.

Blood vessels and lymphatics of the pharynx

The blood supply is derived from branches of the external carotid artery:

- Ascending pharyngeal artery
- Facial artery via ascending palatine and tonsillar arteries
- Maxillary artery via greater palatine and pterygoid arteries
- Lingual artery

To remember these just think of 'MALF' – maxillary, ascending pharyngeal/palatine, lingual and facial. Veins drain into submucosal and external pharyngeal venous plexuses which drain to the internal jugular vein.

Lymphatics drain to the deep cervical nodes.

Nerve supply to the pharynx

Motor: The glossopharyngeal nerve (cranial nerve IX) supplies stylopharyngeus while all the other pharyngeal muscles are supplied by the vagus nerve (cranial nerve X) through its pharyngeal branch to the pharyngeal plexus.

In truth the pharyngeal branch of the vagus is transmitting cranial accessory (cranial nerve XI) nerve fibres that join the vagus nerve in the jugular foramen.

Sensory: Nasopharynx – maxillary nerve (Part 2 of trigeminal nerve – V_2) and glossopharyngeal nerve (CN IX)

Oropharynx – CN IX

Laryngopharynx – internal laryngeal nerve (CN X)

This is probably the most complex part of the physiology to remember so read this again.

Anatomy and physiology of the larynx

The larynx is the organ of phonation. Speech is one of the characteristics which has given humans a selective advantage over other species and is dependant on an adequate expiratory air stream from the lungs, tension of the vocal folds to generate the fundamental voice frequency, the articulatory muscle activity of the palate, tongue and lips aided by the resonance characteristics of the nasopharynx, nose and sinuses.

It may help to recall this if you can think of playing a woodwind instrument such as the recorder. There are three components: first, the respiratory pump from your lungs for both speech and the recorder; second, the fundamental tone generator, the larynx for speech or the recorder in this example; third, the modulators, how you position the tongue, lips etc for different speech sounds or your fingers to occlude the holes on the recorder and alter the sound.

The larynx is one of the constriction points of the respiratory system and serves to protect and separate the respiratory system from the digestive system. The cough reflex is one of the lower airway protective mechanisms in which the larynx plays a role. The larynx is important in increasing intra-abdominal pressure by fixing the diaphragm – when you take a deep breath and close your glottis by vocal cord contraction (so the air doesn't escape) – and is used in defecation, micturition and parturition.

A diagram of the larynx is shown below. You ought to be able to name the parts shown, and with the exception of the epiglottis all are either visible or palpable on neck examination.

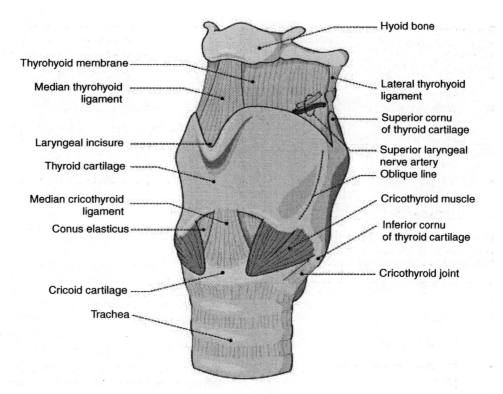

Figure 3.2 Diagram of the larynx

Median cricothyroid ligament or membrane is an important landmark for emergency cricothyroidotomy to gain airway access in upper airway obstruction eg epiglottitis.

You should try to remember the following diagram as it is what you will see when you have an endoscopic view of the larynx.

Also, you will have to be able to describe pathology when you see it. The ventricular folds (aka vestibular folds, false vocal cords) have little role in normal phonation and more in protection.

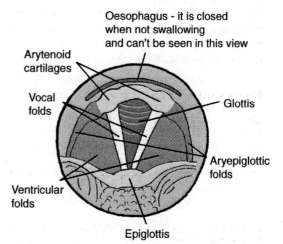

Figure 3.3 Diagram of an endoscopic view of the top of the larynx. (Reproduced with permission from the Lions Voice Clinic, University of Minnesota. Available at: www.lionsvoiceclinic.umn.edu/page2. htm#anatomy101)

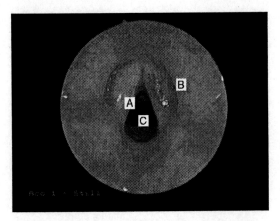

Figure 3.4 Endoscopic view of the larynx. A is left vocal fold, B is right aryepiglottic fold, C is tracheal lumen. (Library property of DA Nunez)

The larynx is divided into three regions.

- Supraglottis – the region above the vocal folds
- Glottis – the level of the vocal folds
- Subglottis – the region below the vocal folds

The supraglottis is the region above the vocal folds that consists of the epiglottis, aryepiglottic folds and laryngeal ventricles.

The level of the vocal folds that includes the vocal processes of the arytenoid cartilages and the space between the vocal folds (narrowed on phonation) is called the glottis.

The region below is the subglottis and extends to the lower border of the cricoid before continuing as the trachea.

These regions are important for describing pathological findings and because the lymphatic drainage is different. There is no direct lymphatic drainage to the cervical lymph nodes from the glottis but good drainage from the supra and sub glottis.

Laryngeal muscles

Figure 3.5 shows an axial view of the muscles and cartilage of the larynx.

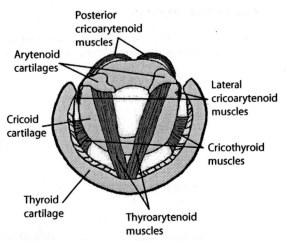

Figure 3.5 Diagram of laryngeal muscles (Reproduced with permission from the Lions Voice Clinic, University of Minnesota. Available at: www.lionsvoiceclinic.umn.edu/page2.htm#anatomy101)

The laryngeal muscles are classified as intrinsic or extrinsic. Intrinsic muscles originate and are inserted onto the laryngeal cartilages. Extrinsic laryngeal muscles either originate or are inserted onto structures besides the laryngeal cartilages.

There are four paired intrinsic laryngeal muscles labelled in the figure only one of which (cricothyroid) does not attach to the arytenoid cartilage. The inter-arytenoid muscle (not shown) runs posteriorly between the two arytenoid cartilages. The epiglottic muscles thyroepiglottic and aryepiglottic are extensions of the thyroarytenoid and interarytenoid muscles respectively into the aryepiglottic folds.

The extrinsic laryngeal muscles elevate or depress the larynx and include the midline strap muscles sterno-thyroid, sterno-hyoid and thyro-hyoid. All muscles that attach to the hyoid bone include: mylo-hyoid, genio-hyoid, omo-hyoid, stylo-hyoid and the digastric. The pharyngeal muscles that are attached to the thyroid cartilage (stylopharyngeus, palatopharyngeus and the inferior constrictor) play a role in stabilising or mobilising the larynx and also belong to the group of extrinsic laryngeal muscles.

Again, this is complicated. Please re-read it until you are happy you understand this.

Laryngeal nerves

There are two rules to learn about the function and innervation of the intrinsic laryngeal muscles. These are:

1. **All** of the intrinsic laryngeal muscles **ADDuct** the vocal cords, **except:**

    The **posterior cricoarytenoid muscle,** which is an ABDuctor

2. **All** of the intrinsic laryngeal muscles are innervated by the **recurrent laryngeal nerve, except:**

    The **cricothyroid muscle,** that is innervated by the **external laryngeal nerve** (a branch of the superior laryngeal nerve)

The laryngeal mucosa is ciliated columnar respiratory in type with the exception of the upper posterior half of the epiglottis, upper aryepiglottic surfaces, the vocal fold membranes and the lining of the posterior interarytenoid space.

Autopsy laryngeal studies suggest that areas of squamous metaplasia occur in the subglottis even in adult nonsmokers. The mucosa is loosely attached to the underlying structures except over the vocal folds, where it is tightly adherent. Taste glands are present on the posterior upper half of the epiglottis and the aryepiglottic folds. Mucous secreting glands are predominantly found on the posterior epiglottis and on the undersurface of the vestibular folds. There are microvilli and ridges on the epithelial surface of the vocal folds.

Larynx blood vessels and lymphatics

The larynx is receives its blood supply from

*   the superior laryngeal artery (a branch of the superior thyroid artery) and

*   the inferior laryngeal artery (a branch of the inferior thyroid artery).

Venous drainage is via the superior and middle laryngeal veins into the internal jugular and the inferior laryngeal vein into the brachiocephalic vein.

There is no direct lymphatic drainage to the cervical lymph nodes from the glottis but good drainage from the supra and sub glottis. The subglottic lymph drainage follows the inferior laryngeal vessels, while the supraglottic follows the superior laryngeal vessels. Therefore neck node metastases are relatively early from laryngeal cancers that originate above or below the vocal folds and can predate the onset of hoarseness. Vocal fold laryngeal cancers on the other hand most usually present with a hoarse voice before the onset of neck swelling related to cervical lymphadenopathy.

Clinical history

In taking a history from a patient presenting with a throat complaint the main questions to ask are related to:

*   Sore throat
*   Dysphonia (hoarseness of the voice)
*   Dysphagia (difficulty in swallowing)
*   Stridor
*   Referred otalgia

Associated questions include:

*   Occupation eg singer, school teacher
*   Smoking habits
*   Alcohol habits
*   Weight loss
*   Heartburn

Dysphonia (hoarseness of voice)

Hoarseness lasting longer than three weeks is a laryngeal carcinoma unless proved otherwise. This is important. Questions to ask are the onset and duration of the hoarseness, whether it is persistent or intermittent, the severity of it, and if there are any trigger factors eg an upper respiratory tract infection. Additionally, ask about systemic symptoms, associated weight loss, smoking and alcohol history, and dysphagia. General medical history is also important, for example neurological problems such as motor neurone disease or myasthenia gravis. Ask about neck lumps. As with everything, observe the patient's mental state – anxiety can cause pseudo-paralysis of the vocal cord adductor. This is commoner in young women.

Dysphagia (difficulty in swallowing)

Questions to ask include the onset and duration of the dysphagia, whether it is painful or painless, intermittent or progressive. Can you swallow liquids or not? Do you ever regurgitate food? Weight loss, reflux, alcohol and smoking history should also be obtained.

Stridor

Stridor is a wheezing type noise created due to turbulent airflow through a narrowing of the larynx (or trachea). This is a very important symptom, especially in children and requires emergency intervention. Stridor should be contrasted with stertor the term used to describe noise secondary to partial obstruction in the pharynx or oral cavity. This is more dissonant in character and can be described as gurgling. The history in both situations needs to include onset, trauma, any infections, inhaled foreign bodies, neurological problems and the relationship to the phase of respiration (inspiratory, expiratory or both).

Clinical examination

Examination of the larynx, nasopharynx and hypopharynx are specialist skills and are unlikely to be assessed in a medical student OSCE, but you have to know how to inspect the oral cavity and oropharynx.

The best thing to do after introduction and permission is to inspect the oral cavity using a tongue depressor and bright torch. Examine the condition of the tongue, look to see if it is deviated, twitching, wasted etc. Ask the patient to move the tongue from one side to the other and inspect not only the dorsum of the tongue but the sides and the under surface (ask the patient to touch the tip of the tongue to their hard palate to allow this area to be inspected). Inspect the floor of the mouth when the tongue is elevated, look for swellings in the submandibular ducts as they run forward to open adjacent to the lingual frenulum. Inspect the gums, teeth and mucosal surfaces of the cheeks. Are there any white (leukoplakia) or red (erythroplakia) patches?

If you press down on the tongue with a tongue depressor you can examine the back of the **tongue** and the **tonsils,** as well as the uvula and soft palate. See Figure 3.6 below which shows you the structures:

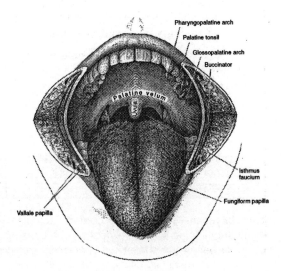

Figure 3.6 View of the oral cavity
Gray H (1918) Anatomy of the Human Body,
20th edition, Lea & Febiger, Philadelphia
(This image is in the public domain because its copyright has expired. This applies worldwide.)

Next you ought to inspect the hard palate by asking the patient to tip their head back. Use the tongue depressor to gently retract the mucosa of the cheek from the gums to allow inspection of the mucosa between the cheeks and gums – the gingivo-buccal sulcus and the parotid duct opening.

Diseases of the throat

This will cover hoarseness of the voice, sore throat and stridor.

Hoarse voice

The patient describes a change in the quality of the voice usually involving the pitch, and or volume of the speaking or singing voice. This can be due to pathology anywhere along the voice production pathway. The latter consists of the lungs and chest that produce the expiratory air drive, the vocal folds that generate the fundamental speech frequency

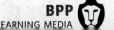

as the expired air passes through the glottis, and the actions of the soft palate and tongue that modify the resonance.

Therefore disease affecting expiratory lung volume, the lining of the vocal folds or neurolomuscular function may have an impact on clear phonation.

The causes can be divided into local (vocal fold), neurological and muscular.

Local causes (common causes in bold):

- **Upper respiratory tract infection**
- **Laryngitis**
- **Voice overuse**
- Vocal fold polyps
- Vocal nodules
- Pharyngeal acid reflux
- Laryngeal carcinoma
- Lung cancer
- Thyroid cancer
- Oesophageal cancer
- Trauma
- Hypothyroidism

Neurological causes:

- Laryngeal nerve palsy (including iatrogenic eg thyroid surgery, cardiac surgery)
- Motor neurone disease (MND)
- Myasthenia gravis

Muscular causes:

- Muscular dystrophy (rare)

Other causes include cricoarytenoid joint arthritis, which may be caused by:

- Rheumatoid arthritis
- Gout
- Systemic lupus erythematosus (SLE)

Treatment depends upon diagnosis of the cause and this is usually achieved by a full history, examination and usually inspection with a fibreoptic scope.

Laryngeal cancer

Histologically primary cancer of the larynx consists of dysplastic change of the epithelial lining with spread through the underlying basement membrane. Cancer of the larynx is overwhelmingly squamous cell carcinoma and primary rather than due to secondary spread. Secondary involvement is usually due to direct spread from the adjacent pharynx or thyroid. Laryngeal carcinoma is the second commonest malignancy of the head and neck after squamous cell carcinoma of the skin in this region. The condition affects males more than females 9:1 and has a peak incidence in the 7th–8th decade. Tobacco smoking and alcohol consumption are the main aetiological factors.

A persistent hoarse voice is the commonest presenting complaint. Pain is not a frequent presenting feature but a few patients present with referred otalgia when there is pharyngeal spread. You may recall that sensation from the pharynx and larynx is transmitted through the pharyngeal plexus with input from the glossopharyngeal and sensory component of the vagus nerves. These nerves also supply the deep external auditory meatus thus providing a pathway for referred otalgia in relation to primary pathology in the hypopharynx.

Examination must include, in addition to laryngeal inspection with fibreoptic laryngoscopy, palpation of the neck to document cervical lymphadenopathy.

Investigation protocols differ between institutions, but in many will include full blood count and serum electrolytes as these patients can be anaemic and dehydrated if disease is extensive, and liver function tests because of the strong association with high alcohol intake and to exclude metastases to the liver. CT scan of the head, neck and chest is also required to help with local staging and exclude lung and brain metastases (or in the case of the lung a synchronous primary cancer of the lower respiratory tract). Synchronous aerodigestive tract cancers occur in 10% of cases. The liver is imaged either by ultrasound or by extending the CT scan field to include the abdomen.

Tissue diagnosis is imperative and is obtained by direct laryngoscopy in the operating room. Treatment depends on patient factors, especially co-morbidity, and disease factors, mostly the extent of the disease and available clinical expertise. All of these are taken into consideration by clinicians when making treatment decisions in the multidisciplinary team (MDT) in the UK, or tumour board meeting in North America.

Two cancer-staging systems commonly used in making treatment decisions are the American Joint Cancer Committee (AJCC) and the Union International Contre le Cancer (UICC). In both, laryngeal cancers are staged on the basis of local tumour extent (T stage), neck lymph node involvement (N stage) and the presence of distant metastasis (M stage). Early disease will not demonstrate nodal, distant metastases or have much local extension. In the case of a cancer of the vocal cord, only one part of one vocal cord may be involved without reducing the movement of the vocal cord, defined as T1 disease in both systems. The other extreme will be a T4 cancer, graded as such because it extends beyond the confines of the larynx itself either by invading through the laryngeal cartilages or growing into the pharynx. A patient with a T4 tumour will have nodal involvement and in a proportion distant metastasis.

In early stage disease, the current trend in North America and the UK is to undertake microlaryngoscopic guided CO_2 laser resection. In advanced disease, treatment can be chemoradiotherapy, surgery (laryngectomy with or without neck dissection) or surgery followed by chemoradiotherapy. A total laryngectomy requires the removal of the larynx with the tracheal airway below the resection being anastomosed to the skin at the front of neck that is fashioned into a **tracheostoma** (see Figure 3.7). The subtotal types of laryngectomy are not be discussed in this text. The patient breathes through the post laryngectomy stoma but normal speech is lost.

A number of techniques have been developed to overcome this handicap. Oesophageal speech requires the patient to learn how to expel swallowed air past the reconstructed cricopharyngeus (upper oesophageal) sphincter thus recreating the three components of the speech production pathway as described previously. A speaking valve can be placed through the posterior tracheal wall to create a one-way fistula into the upper oesophagus (trachea-oesophageal puncture). The patient then directs expired air from the lungs by occluding the tracheostoma with their hand into the oesophagus via the valve. The action of the cricopharyngeus on the expired air replaces the function of the larynx.

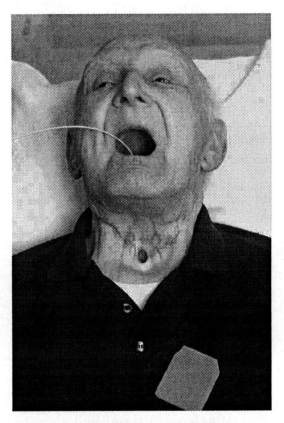

Figure 3.7 Post laryngectomy tracheostoma displayed in patient undergoing balloon oesophageal dilation. (Reproduced courtesy of Vaghela HM et al. _Journal of Laryngology & Otology_ (2006), 120, 56–58.)

Benign conditions that cause hoarseness

Vocal fold nodules

This is a condition classically seen in boys under the age of 10 and is caused by secondary changes in the vocal folds related to shouting. Professional voice users, for example teachers or telephone receptionists are at risk. The diagnosis is made by laryngoscopy when symmetrical swellings of the vocal folds at the junction of the anterior 2/3 and posterior 1/3 is seen. The mainstay of treatment is speech therapy but surgical removal is sometimes required.

Vocal fold polyps

These present in adults – usually smokers and singers. There is symmetrical oedematous enlargement of the vocal folds which presents as vocal fold polyps. Diagnostic microlaryngoscopy and biopsy is required to exclude laryngeal cancer. A number of microlaryngoscopic techniques, beyond the scope of this text, exist to manage this condition. Avoidance of the predisposing factors is essential if a recurrence is to be avoided.

Sore throat

A sore throat is the main presenting symptom of pharyngitis. This is exceptionally common and a list of differentials must be in your head. In the UK, a general practitioner with about 2,000 patients sees approximately 120 cases per year, some of which need investigation.

Common causes of pharyngitis are:

Infectious

- Viral
    - Rhinovirus (common cold)
    - Epstein-Barr (infectious mononucleosis or glandular fever)
    - Influenza
    - Acquired immune deficiency
- Bacterial
    - Streptococcus
    - Tonsillitis
    - Peritonsillar abscess (quinsy)
- Fungal
    - Candida albicans

Non-infectious

- Acid reflux
- Trauma
- Malignancy

In addition to odynophagia (pain on swallowing), the history consists of fever, headache, nausea, vomiting, abdominal pain, rhinorrhoea, post-nasal drip, heart-burn, foul breath or weight loss depending on the cause.

Investigations may include a throat swab (most infections are viral), and even antigen testing. The mainstay of treatment is analgesia, antipyretics, fluids and gargling with salt water.

Antibiotics are not usually indicated in the majority of adult patients with sore throat. When antibiotics are required in the management of bacterial pharyngitis the possibility of infectious mononucleosis should be excluded before prescribing amoxicillin because of the risk of widespread skin rash.

Tonsillectomy is indicated in the management of frequent episodes of recurrent tonsillitis, that is, six or more episodes per year for two or more years, to reduce the impact of the condition on the patients and their carers' lives.

Glandular fever (infectious mononucleosis) caused by the Epstein-Barr virus is suggested by bilateral tonsillar enlargement and prominent cervical adenopathy presenting in young adulthood or late adolescence. Look for more systemic symptoms and signs eg hepatosplenomegaly, rash, jaundice, widespread adenopathy, elevated liver enzymes and lymphocytosis. Treatment is with bed rest, fluids, paracetamol (acetaminophen), steroids, antibiotics for secondary infections and alcohol abstinence. Contact sports should be avoided particularly if there are signs of hepatosplenomegaly.

Complications of bacterial pharyngitis and tonsillitis include:

- Peritonsillar abscess (quinsy)
- Retropharyngeal abscess
- Other parapharyngeal abscesses
- Rheumatic fever
- Glomerulonephritis

The first two are common and can present with the initial attack of tonsillitis. Retropharyngeal abscess is seen almost exclusively in young children and peritonsillar abscess from late adolescence throughout adulthood.

Stridor

Note the definition and history of stridor as described in the *Clinical history* section above. Causes are:

Congenital

- Laryngomalacia
- Subglottic haemanagioma
- Bilateral vocal fold paralysis

Accquired

- Subglottic stenosis
- Inhaled foreign body
- Croup (laryngotracheobronchitis)
- Laryngeal paralysis
- Epiglottitis (usually now seen primarily in adults)
- Trauma (eg laryngeal fracture)

The signs are:

- Inspiratory wheeze (however this depends on where the laryngeal airway is restricted. It can be heard from the other end of the room)

- Tachypnoea

- Use of accessory muscles of respiration

- Tracheal tug

- Pallor

- Cyanosis

Treat the cause after doing ABC.

Epiglottitis

This is a potentially life-threatening bacterial infection causing inflammation (oedema, erythema) of the epiglottis and adjacent upper laryngeal structures. Prior to the introduction of the Haemophilus influenza B vaccine, this was a condition seen primarily in children secondary to Haemophilus influenza type B infection. Nowadays the condition is more commonly seen in adults, (check their immunisation status) and is caused by beta haemolytic Streptococcus or H. influenza.

Symptoms are:

- Sore throat especially on swallowing
- Dysphagia
- Stridor
- Drooling
- Fever
- Shortness of breath
- Restlessness

If you suspect the diagnosis in children, **do not** undertake a detailed examination of the oral cavity, pharynx or larynx without facilities for intubation or tracheotomy, because fatal laryngospasm or mucus plugging of the airway can be triggered. Examination of the pharynx and larynx should only take place in the hospital operating theatre with access to full resuscitation including tracheostomy equipment.

In adults the presentation is less dramatic with stridor being both less common and prominent. A thorough examination of the adult patient's pharynx and larynx can be undertaken in the ward or emergency department usually with a flexible laryngoscope as the risks of losing the airway is insignificant. It is more characteristic to see diffuse oedema of the upper laryngeal structures rather than exclusively the epiglottis. The condition is therefore sometimes referred to as supraglottitis.

Treatment is with intravenous steroids, antibiotics (as this is a bacterial infection in contradistinction to croup where the infection is viral) and close observation. Airway intubation and ICU admission is usually required in children but rarely in adults who can be managed in a high dependency environment. Tracheostomy is seldom undertaken nowadays.

Neck

To be comfortable with understanding neck pathology you ought to be confident with your anatomy. The anatomy of the neck (with regard to ENT) will be discussed initially. We then go on to consider questions to ask in a neck history, look at how to conduct a neck examination and, finally, explore specific pathologies.

Anatomy of the neck

To be able to describe the location of neck lumps, the neck is divided into several parts based upon certain anatomical landmarks. Figure 3.8 shows the main divisions of the neck.

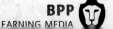

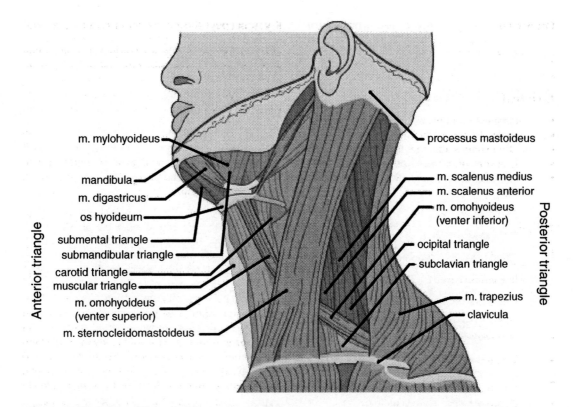

Figure 3.8 Triangular divisions of the neck

Thus, it is the sternocleidomastoid muscle (SCM) that is the main muscular landmark, which bisects the neck diagonally into the anterior and posterior cervical (neck) triangles, as shown above.

The borders of the anterior triangle of the neck are as follows:

- Anterior: midline of the neck

- Posterior: anterior border of sternocleidomastoid muscle

- Superior (base of triangle): inferior border of the mandible

- Inferior (apex of triangle): suprasternal (jugular) notch

The borders of the posterior triangle of the neck are as follows:

- Anterior: posterior border of sternocleidomastoid muscle

- Posterior: anterior border of trapezius

- Superior (apex of triangle): union of sternocleidomastoid muscle and trapezius at the occiput

- Inferior (base of triangle): middle third of the claricle

The contents of the triangles should be revised. The importance of this will be better understood when diagnoses are discussed below.

First however, it is necessary to discuss the arrangement of lymph nodes in the neck. They are arranged as follows:

Anterior triangle

Level 1	Submental and submandibular
Level 2	Upper deep cervical
Level 3	Middle deep cervical
Level 4	Lower deep cervical

Posterior triangle

Level 5	Posterior triangle
Level 6	Paratracheal lymph nodes
Level 7	Mediastinal nodes

We will now consider how to take a history from someone who presents with a neck lump, and what the key questions are.

Clinical history

When someone presents with a neck lump, several factors have to be taken into account. These include the patient's age, sex, local symptoms, and smoking and alcohol habits as a general inquiry. More specific questions about the neck lump ought to include:

- Site?
- Onset?
- Change in size, shape and colour?
- Is it tender? Red?
- Has there been any discharge?
- Has it been there a long time, or appeared recently?
- Enquire about symptoms resulting from local causes of lymphadenopathy eg dysphagia, otorrhoea, rhinorrhea, aryngitis, dyspnoea and referred otalgia.
- Systemic questions such as sweating/fevers, drug/sexual/travel history for infectious causes, pain with drinking alcohol and symptoms of thyroid pathology (bowel habit, temperature sensitivity, menstrual irregularity etc).

The above is a general outline, and when discussing each specific disease, more detail will be given.

Clinical examination

The key to examining neck lumps is to follow the basic principles of clinical examination. Obtain the patient's consent and follow with:

- Exposure
- Inspection
- Palpation
- Percussion
- Auscultation

Percussion, you may think, what for? But it is important, and each of the above will be considered separately.

Exposure

You have to get complete exposure of the head and neck down to the clavicles, and get the patient to sit comfortably in a chair.

Inspection

The key to diagnosis is inspection. Inspection of the area around the patient is important, as it may give you clues, eg a glass of water next to the patient may indicate that they do not have a problem swallowing.

On inspection look for evidence of hypo/ hyperthyroidism and any obvious abnormalities or scars. Look behind the ears also. You can ask the patient to swallow and see if any masses move (you'll understand why later). Is there a midline swelling? Ask the patient to stick out their tongue and see if it moves with the tongue. How does their facial nerve appear to be functioning? Can they screw up their eyes, show you their teeth etc, as a parotid tumour may disrupt facial nerve function (remember – in the parotid, CN VII divides into temporal, zygomatic, buccal, maxillary and cervical branches). Is there any lid lag – hyperthyroidism?

Ask the patient to count from 1 to 20 to see if there is any problem with his voice, implying recurrent laryngeal nerve problems (for example, due to thyroid pathology/previous surgery).

Then assess the following characteristics of any lumps:

- Position
- Size
- Shape
- Consistency
- Fixation
- Colour
- Tenderness
- Movement with swallowing (mentioned above)

Palpation

Palpation is very important as it allows you to ascertain much information about the lump.

You should ideally palpate the whole neck, but don't spend too long on everywhere and try to focus on the lump you have identified on inspection. Stand behind the patient and explain to them what you are about to do. Then put both your hands under their jaw and move from the midline laterally with your fingers 'walking' up the side of their mandible. Then go up behind their ears (pre and postauricular lymph nodes), down along the SCM feeling deep to it and hence palpating the nodes all the way down it to the paratracheal (either side of the trachea) and then into the posterior triangle.

If you identify a lump, check if it is fluctuant, fixed to skin or to deeper structures, pulsatile and if it can be transilluminated.

Try to observe an ENT surgeon and then practise these techniques for yourself. It gets easier with time.

Figure 3.9 (below) shows lymphatics in the neck.

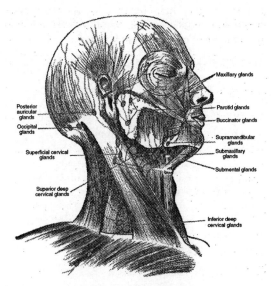

Figure 3.9 Lymphatics in the neck
Gray H (1918) Anatomy of the Human Body,
20th edition, Lea & Febiger, Philadelphia
(This image is in the public domain because its copyright has expired. This applies worldwide.)

Percussion

This is important in examining thyroid pathology. You can percuss over the manubrium sternum for retrosternal goitre. When it enlarges it can get all the way back there, thus it is worth a check.

Auscultation

The main structures in the neck that you can auscultate are the thyroid gland and the carotid arteries. Listen over the thyroid because if the thyroid is large and hypervascular then a bruit may be heard. Listen over the carotids for a bruit, but beware that aortic stenosis may radiate there also. Plus, it may be occluded so much that there may be no flow sound.

Diseases of the neck

Neck pathology usually presents as a new lump in the neck. As with most other pathology it may be congenital or acquired. Congenital causes include:

- Cystic hygroma
- Branchial cyst
- Thyroglossal cyst

To aid diagnosis neck lumps will be described with respect to their commonest location in the neck eg midline, anterior triangle and posterior triangle. In patients under 20 years of age the cause is usually congenital or infection. In the 20–40 year old age range lymphomas should be added to the common differential diagnoses. In the over 40s, metastatic carcinoma **must** always be presumed.

Midline lumps

Lumps in the midline may be arising from the thyroid gland, its developmental pathway as in a thyroglossal cyst or the skin (eg a dermoid cyst). Dermoid cysts and sebaceous cysts may of course occur anywhere.

Thyroid swellings

These can be classified as follows:

1. Diffuse goitre
2. Multinodular goitre
3. Solitary thyroid nodule

Diffuse goitre

This condition is a non-toxic diffuse enlargement of the whole gland. There is no associated nodularity and it is not associated with hypo or hyperthyroidism. It is a compensatory hypertrophy and hyperplasia secondary to a reduction in T3 and/or T4 output (and hence driven by an increase in thyroid stimulating hormone (TSH)).

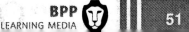

Diffuse goitres can revert to normal, stay the same or develop into a multinodular goitre.

The aetiology is as follows:

- Physiological – increased demand for thyroid hormone such as puberty or pregnancy
- Dietary – iodine deficiency – the commonest cause by far worldwide
- Hereditary
- Treated Grave's disease – if Grave's is untreated then the patient would be thyrotoxic yet these patients are euthyroid
- Hashimoto's thyroiditis
- Reidel's thyroiditis

Multinodular goitre

Multinodular goitres are just that, on examination and/or investigation, the enlargement consists of several nodules. They can be toxic or non-toxic.

Aetiology:

Non-toxic

- Progression from diffuse goitre – the commonest cause. These have areas of multinodular focal hyperplasia.
- Sporadic multinodular goitre
- Rare syndromes – Pendred syndrome – an inherited syndrome associated with hearing loss

Toxic

- Grave's disease

Solitary thyroid nodule

These can either be a palpable true solitary nodule, a prominent nodule in an otherwise multinodular goitre, or a non-palpable nodule diagnosed as an incidental finding on a utrasound or other imaging investigation. Palpable thyroid nodules can be found in approximately 5% of the population and on high-resolution ultrasound scanning in more than 50%. The majority, 90–95%, of solitary nodules are benign or, put another way, 5%–10% are malignant.

The main question to be answered when encountering a thyroid nodule is to determine if it is malignant or not. The common investigations are thyroid function blood tests to determine if the patient is euthyroid or otherwise; thyroid autoantibodies; ultrasound thyroid scan, and fine needle aspiration cytology (FNAC).

Thyroid cancer

Primary thyroid epithelial cancer is classified into four histological types:

- Papillary
- Follicular
- Medullary
- Anaplastic

Papillary thyroid cancer

This is the commonest type and affects young people (30–40 years of age) with a slight female predominance 2:1. It has a good prognosis generally (ten-year survival approximately 90%). Treatment is usually thyroid lobectomy for small tumours and total thyroidectomy for large tumours (>1cm). It can also include lymph node neck dissection usually level 6. Most patients will also undergo radioiodine thyroid ablation.

These tumours are TSH dependent and hence all patients need high dose thyroxine for life (to suppress TSH and hence tumour recurrence).

Follicular thyroid cancer

These are the second commonest type, and typically present in females in their fifties. They cannot be distinguished from benign follicular adenomas on FNAC. Evidence of a follicular neoplasm on FNAC requires a diagnostic thyroid lobectomy for histology. Treatment for follicular carcinoma includes completion thyroidectomy, neck lymph node dissection, radioiodine thyroid ablation and post-operative thyroxine.

Medullary thyroid cancer

These cancers originate from the parafollicular C cells (that make calcitonin). The majority arise de-novo but up to one-third are hereditary – either familial medullary thyroid cancer or multiple endocrine neoplasia syndrome. The prognosis is less than 50% five-year survival but not as poor as anaplastic cancers. It presents equally in males and females. Surgery, namely total thyroidectomy and neck dissection, is the mainstay of treatment as these tumours are not responsive to radioiodine and thyroid hormone suppression.

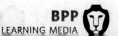

Anaplastic

This is the most aggressive kind of cancer. It presents in the elderly with a woody thyroid and compressive neck symptoms. Patients usually require palliative care with this type of thyroid cancer. The prognosis is poor with survival from diagnosis measured usually in months. Palliative thyroidectomy may be required along with tracheostomy to secure the airway.

To prepare for a thyroid case in your end of year or rotation assessments you should master the clinical neck examination routine. You also need to be familiar with some of the facts described to allow you to come to a sensible diagnosis and interpret the findings with respect to the above causes.

Thyroglossal cyst

This arises from remnant of the thyroglossal duct, which traces the embryological path of the thyroid from the tongue base (foramen ceacum) to its final position in the neck. It classically occurs between the level of the hyoid bone above, and upper border of the thyroid cartilage below, is discrete, midline, round, smooth, non-tender and moves upwards on protruding the tongue. Surgical removal in continuity with the middle third of the hyoid bone is the recommended treatment (Sistrunk's procedure).

Dermoid cyst

These present as mobile, smooth and cutaneous swellings and commonly occur around the eye, nose and in the midline.

Anterior triangle lumps

Branchial cysts, carotid body and parotid tumours are examples.

Branchial cyst

These are centred on the anterior border of the SCM at the junction between the upper 1/3 and lower 2/3. They are believed to be congenital and due to remnants of the cervical sinus of His where the second branchial arch grows over the third and fourth. They present in young adults as a cystic swelling from which cholesterol can be aspirated. It usually enlarges after an upper respiratory tract infection. Treatment is surgical excision.

Carotid body tumour (chemodectoma)

Chemodectomas are rare, but you should know about them. They are slow growing tumours that arise from the chemoreceptor cells in the carotid body, at the carotid artery bifurcation. They are commoner in the over thirties and the most important clinical examination feature is that they are classically pulsatile to palpation. Syncope due to local pressure on the carotid sinus can occur. Check for lower cranial nerve palsies secondary to tumour compression. FNAC of a pulsatile neck mass is not recommended but rather imaging with duplex and MRI or CT scan should be done. Additional investigations include 24-hour urine cathecholamine levels and imaging of the abdomen to exclude adrenal tumours. Treatment can be conservative or surgical excision. These tumours are not radiosensitive.

Parotid pathology

The commonest (benign) parotid lesion is the **pleomorphic adenoma**. These can present at any age as a slow growing swelling anywhere in the parotid, most commonly near the angle of the mandible in the tail of the parotid gland. The clinical features would be a well-defined, firm non-tender lump. In the patient with a parotid swelling, always examine the mouth and oropharynx to see if there is any swelling of the ipsilateral buccal mucosa that may represent calculus obstruction of the parotid duct, generalised swelling of the gland (due to parotitis) or medial displacement of the tonsil (indicative of a deep lobe parotid or other parapharyngeal tumour). Complete the neck examination checking for regional lymph nodes to exclude metastases. Facial nerve function should be assessed and is always intact unless the tumour is malignant.

FNAC is the main investigation. Treatment is parotidectomy with facial nerve preservation. Pleomorphic adenomas left untreated for 10–15 years can become malignant, carcinoma ex-pleomorphic adenoma.

Posterior triangle lumps

These include lymph node swellings and cystic hygroma.

Lymph node swellings may be due to malignancy or infection (HIV/TB) so take a full history. When examining lymph nodes think of lymph drainage and where a primary lesion may be. Level 1 to 4 is usually due to the tongue, other midline throat structures and the floor of the mouth. Posterior triangle lymph nodes eg Level 5 drain the scalp, neck and extra-regional sites such as chest and abdomen (supraclavicular nodes). Pre and post auricular lymph nodes drain from the eye and ear. Think of the local structures that drain into the lymph nodes and that will give you an idea of where the problem may be. Don't forget metastatic skin squamous cell carcinoma presenting as a neck node.

Cystic hygroma

This is a collection of dilated lymph node channels that is found at the base of the posterior triangle and is congenital in nature. It will present in children as a soft fluctuant and compressible lump. It can grow to be so large as to fill the whole of the posterior triangle. It can also be transilluminated, which is an important diagnostic aid. So do shine a torch through any masses in the posterior triangle. It can be treated medically with injection sclerotherapy or surgically.

Investigations of neck lumps

Investigations used in the assessment of neck lumps include ultrasound, fine needle aspiration, virology, and CT/MRI scans.

Red flags in laryngology and neck

- Dysphonia (hoarse voice) – three weeks' duration
- Dysphagia/odynophagia
- Any persistent growing neck lump

What to do in an OSCE

It is important that all of the rudiments of good practice in a clinical setting be followed. These should come naturally to you by the time you are undertaking this type of examination (if you have been diligent in clerking patients in the otolaryngology department).

Therefore do not forgot to introduce yourself to the patient, confirm their identify and obtain consent (usually verbal) to the clinical intervention. If the examination question requires that you take a history from a patient presenting with a throat or neck complaint keep focused on the aim of taking a clinical history, which is to obtain a diagnosis. The junior medical student and even more experienced clinicians can lose sight of this in the artificial setting of an OSCE. The OSCE is not only an exercise in checking if you can recall what questions to ask.

The OSCE question that requires an examination of the patient's head and neck should not be worrisome. Recall the steps of inspection, palpation, percussion and auscultation. Revise the clinical features of the various diagnoses described in this chapter. Be methodical in your approach. It is easy for the novice to forget to palpate part of the neck during an OSCE.

Common areas that students overlook are the parotid region over and in front of the mandibular ramus (while this is actually part of the head or face, a neck examination requires thorough assessment of the major salivary glands) and the posterior triangle region.

When palpating the neck in an otolaryngology OSCE, the aim is to feel the structures deep to the skin and not examine only for lumps that arise from the skin or subcutaneous tissue which would really be part of a dermatology assessment.

References

Cummings CW (2005) *Otolaryngology Head & Neck Surgery*. Vol 3, 4th edition. Philadelphia: Elsevier Mosby.

Costanzo LS (1998) *Physiology*. Philadelphia: Saunders.

Fry J and Sandler G (1993) *Common diseases: their nature, presentation and care*. 5th edition. Lancaster: Kluwer Academic Publishers. pp. 66–73.

Lions Voice Clinic. *About the Voice* [Online] Available at: www.lionsvoiceclinic.umn.edu/page2.htm#anatomy101 [Accessed 08 March 2013].

Mehanna HM et al. Investigating the thyroid nodule. *BMJ* 2009; 21 March vol. 338: 705–709.

Munro JF and Campbell IW (2000) *Macleod's Clinical Examination*. Edinburgh: Churchill Livingstone.

Scottish Intercollegiate Guidelines Network. *Management of Sore Throat and Indications for Tonsillectomy* [Online] Available at: www.sign.ac.uk/pdf/sign117.pdf [Accessed 11 August 2011].

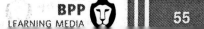

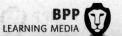

Chapter 4

Facial plastic surgery

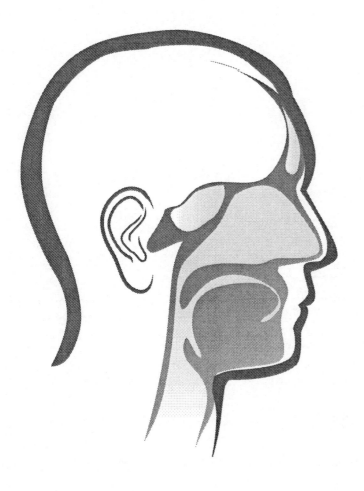

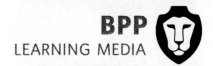

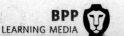

Introduction

'Beauty is in the eye of the beholder' has been a common theme for artists and their subjects alike. The art work which has been preserved from era to era and civilisation to civilisation illustrates what was considered to be the 'ideal' beauty of that time. Stone carvings dating back to the Palaeolithic era display the human form as art. The basic anthropological principle: human features deemed attractive change with time, but the social, reproductive, and evolutionary advantages they convey do not. These fundamental facts provide the driving force for the development of facial cosmetic surgery as an emerging and ever changing specialty within the practice of medicine. The human face acts as a canvas upon which many different scenes can be played out, furthering man's attempt to reach the ideal human form. The ideal human form of course varies significantly across time, from generation to generation, and millennium to millennium. Ethnicity plays a significant role in what each civilisation considers the ideal human and facial form.

The very word aesthetic is derived from the Greek 'aesthesis' meaning to have sense of or devotion to beauty. The Greek philosophers sought to define ideal beauty with the same mathematical principals and geometric relations that were thought to define the laws of nature. The philosopher Plato who placed great significance on beauty, harmony and mathematic proportions, most likely influenced Greek sculptures whose work was often felt to define the very essence of beauty. It is with this in mind that no discussion of facial cosmetic surgery can be undertaken without the examination of facial proportions.

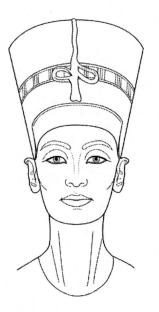

Figure 4.1 Nefertiti

Golden proportion

A significant and interesting mathematical rule of historical significance is known as the golden proportion. This phenomenon was most likely first recognised by the ancient Egyptians, and subsequently adopted by the ancient Greeks. This proportion is not only found in facial identification but also in architecture, which the ancient Greeks viewed as a higher art form and resulted in proportions, which were especially pleasing to the human eye. The golden proportion can be defined as a ratio of two unequal segments of a line, where the ratio of the shorter segment to the longer segment is equal to the ratio of the longest segment to the whole line. The golden proportion is represented by the Greek letter φ and named after the Greek sculptor Phidias (500–432 BC). The actual value of the golden proportion is felt equal to 1.61803.... One example of the golden proportion in analysing the nose is the ratio of nasal projection to nasal length. If this ratio was golden then the nasofacial angle falls within the aesthetic ideal of 36–38 degrees.

Face

As thought by the ancient Greeks, the ideal human head is one-eighth the height of the body and twice the length of the neck. The face can be divided horizontally into thirds on the frontal view. The superior one-third is the forehead from the trichion to the glabella, the middle-third extends from the glabella to the subnasale and the inferior third or the lower portion of the face is the region from the subnasale to the menton (Figure 4.2). Some of these proportions may vary with the change in the hairline.

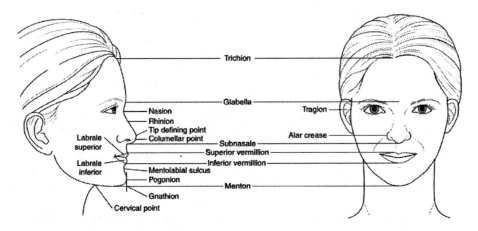

Figure 4.2: The face – some anatomical landmarks

The face can also be divided vertically into equal widths where one eye should be equal to the intercanthal distance, and this width should equal one-fifth of the facial width. Lines from the outer canthi should approximate the width of the neck and the lateral fifth of the face extends from the lateral canthi to the farthest lateral points of the pinna (Figure 4.3).

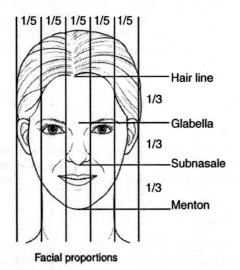

Facial proportions

Figure 4.3 The face divided by vertical lines into equal fifths and horizontal lines into equal thirds

Facial angles

The face is a complex set of curves and contours and, as we may all be aware, extremely variable. One of the primary goals of facial analysis is to be able to evaluate pre-operative and post-operative results. Many of these facial angles are especially important in rhinoplasty patients. One of the most often evaluated facial angle is the 'nasolabial angle' which is defined by the line from the subnasale to the superior vermillion border and the columellar tangent from the subnasale. It is often considered to ideally fall between 90 degrees and 100 degrees in males, and 100 degrees and 110 degrees in females. There are several other facial angles especially important in rhinoplasty including the nasofrontal angle, which is the line connecting the nasion to the glabella and the nasion to the tip-defining point from the nasofrontal angle. This angle should ideally fall between 115–130 degrees. The nasofacial angle is formed by the angle between the facial plane and the line tangent to the nasal dorsum. This angle should be ideally 36–40 degrees. The nasomental angle is formed by the line tangent to the nasal dorsum and the line connecting the tip-defining point of the pogonion. The mento-cervical angle is the line connecting the cervical point of the facial plane to the menton (chin) and should lie between 80 degrees and 95 degrees. Powell and Humphries (1984) incorporated all five facial angles into what they considered the **aesthetic triangle**. This allowed for combining all of the different facial angles and the relations into a single construct for simultaneous evaluation of facial proportions and the independent facial elements.

One important dimension when making facial analysis comparisons especially in the pre-operative and post-operative photographs is the Frankfort plane. This is a horizontal line drawn from the external auditory canal to the inferior orbital rim. This plane represents the neutral position for facial analysis.

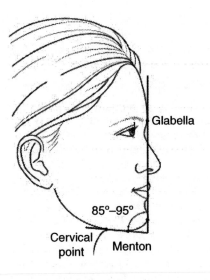

Mento-cervical angle

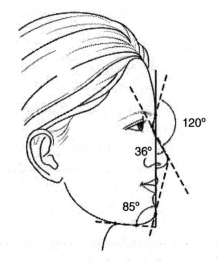

Aesthetic triangle
(Powell and Humphreys)

Figure 4.4: The mento-cervical angle and aesthetic triangle

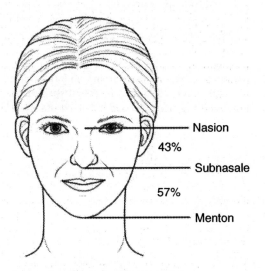

Lower two-thirds facial proportion

Figure 4.5: Facial proportions

The nose

It has been considered by most, that of all the facial aesthetic units, the nose plays the most central role in facial harmony. It has often been said that the fate of many women rests in the shape of their nose. This seems to be even more true now considering the price placed on facial beauty in society ranging from motion pictures to selling cars. The nose is a single unpaired anatomic structure, which occupies the central face and balances the facial thirds and fifths as well as those structures surrounding it. Seemingly small changes to the nose can effect dramatic changes in facial appearance and the other aesthetic units. It is for this reason that we will consider this the first facial subunit to be discussed in detail.

The nose itself can be divided into subunits which can help in pre-operative evaluation and surgical planning of reconstructive and cosmetic procedures. These include:

- Dorsum
- Sidewalls
- Alae
- Tip
- Columella
- Soft-tissue triangles

Nasal anatomy is very complicated. It is important that all of the contituent subunits are considered and addressed if necessary to achieve the desired result of a nasal appearance in harmony with the rest of the face. There are many anatomical components and subcomponents which characterise the nasal anatomy. They are:

- Nasal bone
- Nasomaxillary suture line
- Ascending process of maxilla
- Osseocartilaginous junction (rhinion)
- Upper lateral cartilage
- Anterior septal cartilage
- Caudal free edge of upper lateral cartilage
- Sesamoid cartilage
- Pyriform margin
- Alar lobule
- Lateral crus of alar cartilage – lateral portion
- Lateral crus of alar cartilage – central portion
- Tip – defining point
- Transitional segment of alar cartilage (intermediate crus)
- Infratip lobule
- Columella
- Medial crural footplate

All of these areas and components may be taken into consideration for both pre-operative planning and surgical correction. The rhinoplastic cosmetic surgeon must make themselves familiar with all of these anatomical units.

The philosophy of modern rhinoplasty

The history of modern rhinoplasty surgery and techniques is only about 100 years old. However, in this relatively short period of the surgical time line, many changes have taken place. Initially, the goal was reduction rhinoplasty, that is to make the nose smaller in its appearance. This has changed to become a reconstructive procedure taking into consideration all of the nasal characteristics as well as preservation of function. Within the past two decades, there has been a stronger emphasis on keeping the anatomical proportions of the nose in line with the rest of the patients' facial characteristics. Refinement in techniques combined with better education and improvement in the surgeon's skill have made this a more precise and exacting procedure. Essentially, if a rhinoplasty is performed properly taking into consideration all of the other facial characteristics for the individual patient, the nose itself will look as if the patient was born with it. Ultimately, if done properly, the nose will not draw any particular attention to itself, but blend sinuously with the patient's other natural facial characteristics. If the patient already has a beautiful shaped eye or lips, then the nose should not draw our attention

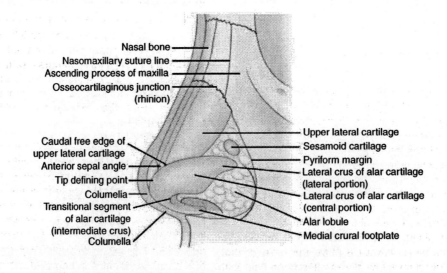

Figure 4.6: Nasal anatomy

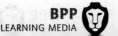

to itself, but allow all of the components and characteristics of the patient's face to shine as one single cosmetic unit.

The 'ideal' nose is not a single entity, where one size fits all. The beauty and facial proportion of the human face varies among the different ethnic groups and is subject to interpretation by each patient as an individual. Much of what patients may consider should be the ideal nose on their face is a combination of several factors including body image and cultural values. This develops from childhood. With the entire world now being connected by satellite, internet, movies, and television the ideal image has changed from culture to culture. What a particular patient's ancestors considered a thing of beauty as a facial characteristic may no longer be viewed by the patient as the ideal. The rhinoplastic surgeon must be sensitive to the patient's own ideals and avoid projecting their own thoughts as to what should be the best cosmetic choice for the patient. Ultimately, it is a combination of these thoughts that may result in the most desired cosmetic result.

Many surgeons operate in areas where there is a single ethnic culture, while more and more, many surgeons are being faced with the difficulties of understanding multiple different cultures. Each surgeon must develop their own artistic concepts and techniques. The surgeon must remember that the nose is the most central portion of the face, but does not stand alone. The best performed rhinoplasties are those that do not look like they were performed at all.

Pre-operative consideration

Many patients will appear in the surgeon's office with a preconceived notion of what the final appearance of the nose should look like. The patients will often bring pictures from magazines of models or famous movie stars as well as pictures of friends. There are times when the nose the patient picks out of a magazine is a realistic consideration, but more times than not, the nose that they see on a movie star's face would not appear natural on their own. This is especially true when their bone structure and other facial features do not support this as a complimentary appearance. This can happen frequently and patients' charts can be replete with pictures they have brought in of magazine covers. Education of the patient by the surgeon and his staff is of the utmost importance

in obtaining a desirable outcome. The patients must be taught that the nose is the central feature of their face and must complement their other facial features in order to look realistic and not 'done'. The conversation often will be basic at first explaining what is realistic in making the nose both cosmetically more desirable as well as retaining nasal function. If the patient still wishes to pursue the intended surgical procedure, a usual process is to then refer them to a photographer who can take a series of views including left, right, downward, and sub-mental vertex, and straight-on views. The patient is asked to come back for an additional consultation with the series of photographs. Slight changes are made on the computer generated images to give the patient an idea of some of the things that can be done. The refining of these pictures takes place during the patient's next consultation with the surgeon.

During the second consultation with the patient's multiple view pictures and computer generated changes, a mirror is utilised so that different areas can be pointed out directly on the patient's own nose. There is usually a back and forth discussion as to what the patient considers ideal and also what the surgeon feels is realistic for both cosmetic beauty and maintaining nasal function. Once the different areas which need to be addressed are agreed upon, notes are made in the patient's chart and on the photographs themselves to ensure that everything that was discussed is addressed during the surgical procedure.

After the patient's consultation, the surgeon must judge whether the patient has realistic motivation and an understanding of the present plan prior to scheduling the desired operation. If there is a doubt in either the patient's or surgeon's mind that the correct procedure will be performed, then a longer period of time may be required to avoid a potential problem.

There are several characteristics that may mark a potential problem patient. Some of these may include unrealistic expectations even after reviewing their own photographs; indecisiveness as to whether they would like to undergo the planned surgical procedure; unco-operativeness in obtaining proper pre-operative photographs or appointments; obsessive-compulsive disorder, and a plastic surgery, 'surgiholic'. Many of these patients have had multiple prior surgical procedures and none of them seem to be satisfactory. The patient is involved in prior litigation against other surgeons. A chronic surgeon shopper is a patient who is disliked by both the surgeon and his staff. Patients who put off all members of staff are difficult to deal with. If any of the above characteristics present themselves, then the surgeon should carefully look at the patient and the planed procedure. There is nothing wrong with a surgeon stating that he does not feel he can make the patient happy and that this would not be a good fit. Remember that a happy patient is one that will go out and spread the word, but one that is unhappy will return over and over again.

Contraindications

Absolute and relative contraindications to rhinoplasty must also be considered. Absolute contraindications to rhinoplasty as in other elective surgery include pregnancy, significant psychiatric and non correctable coagulation disorders. Relative contraindications include temporary or correctable coagulopathies. These patients should be evaluated and pre-treated by a haematologist including specific post-operative instructions and medications. Further relative contraindications include severe nasal acne, psychological disorders (which may not be completely stabilised, but the patient is otherwise functioning) and active autoimmune disease. Some of these may be controlled with medications adequately to allow surgery to proceed, but the possibility of a less than desirable outcome must always be expressed and documented in writing to the patient and in their medical records.

Surgical techniques of rhinoplasty

Rhinoplasty remains one of the most difficult of all plastic facial operations for many reasons. This is a bilateral procedure requiring exacting alteration of bone cartilage and soft tissue components. One of the other most difficult things for the patient and surgeon to understand is that no two cosmetic rhinoplasties are identical just as no two noses are identical – unless of course you have an opportunity to operate on identical twins! Also of great concern is that the surgeon does not have control over the healing process. The ability of the patient's skin to shrink down and take an appropriate contour from the underlying altered nasal support structures is variable. No single surgical technique, no matter how well performed by the surgeon, can prepare the surgeon for the variation in the anatomical patterns and structures of the nose. Therefore, a true rhinoplastic surgeon must be familiar with and trained in many different techniques. Although, he or she may choose one over the other that they are more comfortable with, they must still be able to alter their technique and approach to the one that is most favourable to the individual patient. In many cases of modern rhinoplasty 'less is more'. Rather than over resection and sacrifice large segments of cartilage and bone, the ability to preserve and re-orientate the tissue to develop the desired result will often eliminate large voids of tissue that result in unequal scarring and delayed healing.

In addition to the cosmetic benefits of a more conservative approach, the ability to retain normal nasal function is invariably enhanced leaving more of the supporting structures in place and preventing collapse of the areas of the internal nasal passages such as the nasal valve.

Pre-operative analysis

There are many considerations in the pre-operative analysis, even once the patient and surgeon have agreed upon what they feel would be the desired cosmetic outcome. Each of the nasal subunits must be taken into consideration and appropriate plans made for correcting or not correcting each of these to obtain the desired outcome. The nasal subunits were listed earlier (see *The nose*). Any unnatural over-emphasis of one of these subunits compared to a surrounding subunit may not lend itself to blend gracefully with other areas of the nose. The idea is that all of these units when combined should gracefully blend one into the other and/or not draw particular attention to itself.

During the pre-operative evaluation, the patient's skin must be examined and taken into consideration when planning the procedures to alter the underlying cartilaginous and bony support structures of the nose. There is no ideal skin type which is more favourable in rhinoplasty. Patients of different ethnic backgrounds will all have different types of skin to a greater or lesser extent. The quality and overall thickness of the skin and its supportive subcutaneous tissue exert a major influence on the rhinoplasty procedure and the ultimate outcome. The surgeon uses palpation pre-operatively to judge the skin characteristics, which include thickness, elasticity, and over all quality.

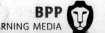

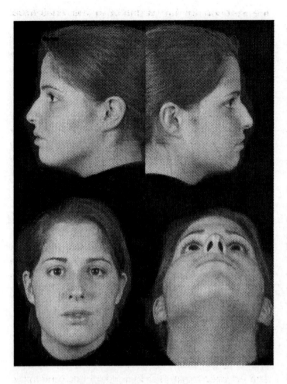

Figure 4.7 Some views used in pre-operative rhinoplasty analysis

After this evaluation, the surgeon can discuss with the patient the overall cosmetic correction that can be achieved. Thin or delicate skin usually develops less post-operative oedema and may heal more quickly. However the skin that is extremely thin or lacking in subcutaneous tissue does not have the ability to camouflage any minor irregularities in the nasal supporting structures. Therefore any slight asymmetric cartilaginous bulge or projection may become readily apparent during the healing process. Thin skin will ultimately allow the rhinoplastic surgeon to achieve more definition, but this must be done carefully and precisely remembering that rhinoplasty is a bilateral procedure.

The patient who has thick skin will tend to heal and contract less quickly. A thick skinned patient will also tend to have greater post-operative oedema. Subcutaneous scar tissue formation may be more abundant and the surgeon who does not take this into consideration will find that he has a greater proportion of patients with an unsightly post-operative polly beak deformity. A polly beak deformity can result from elevation of the cartilaginous dorsum or an overdeveloped vomer. The supra-tip area is elevated and the tip appears amorphous. A post-operative polly beak can result if the dorsal septal cartilage is not adequately resected or in a patient with thick skin.

This is even more common in patients who had had excessive reduction of the nasal dorsum. Smooth redraping of the skin is more difficult when it is thick and therefore the ability to alter and increase definition particularly in the nasal tip may be limited. It may be necessary in these patients to carefully remove some of the subcutaneous tissue to allow better redraping of the skin in the defined tip region. This may also allow a better post-operative contour and definition. However, this must be done with care to prevent scarring in this region or loss of adequate blood supply to the overlying nasal tip skin as this can result in scarring and, if excessive, exposure of the underlying structures. Remember, there is no single best skin type or procedure and the surgeon must be able to consider all of these factors, when planning surgery of the nose.

Selecting an approach for rhinoplasty

The two approaches that are most commonly used for rhinoplasty are the endonasal approach and the open rhinoplasty approach. The bony framework is approached through a combination of inter-cartilaginous incisions, elevation of the skin and soft tissue overlying the dorsum. The dorsum is often reduced first with an osteotome. If the patient does not have a pronounced dorsal hump, this may be reduced slowly with a rasp. The lateral osteotomies can be performed through separate pyriform aperture stab incisions most commonly with a #15 blade. Osteotome selection reflects the surgeon's preference, however a smaller 4mm curved guarded osteotome can work well, where the guarded portion is placed on the medial portion of the nasal bone, thereby leaving areas of undisturbed periosteum on the outer portion of the nasal bone which helps to prevent medial displacement and a more natural appearing contour.

Depending upon how much of the dorsal hump is removed, a medial osteotomy is performed with a 4mm straight unguarded osteotome.

Of primary importance is that the surgeon must be sure that the infracture of each nasal bone is complete. This is often accompanied by a pronounced snap. If the nasal bone is only a 'green-stick' fracture, then over time the nasal bone will again lateralise and the patient will have an asymmetrical nasal dorsum and undesirable cosmetic appearance. If the patient has particularly thick nasal bones especially at the superior extent of the osteotomy, this area can be dealt with directly with a 2mm unguarded osteotome in a small stepwise fashion, which can give a very controlled or complete osteotomy. Some surgeons find this is a difficult region. Again, it should be noted that when elevating the skin and subcutaneous tissue off the dorsum this is not over extended laterally in the region of the future lateral osteotomies. This would be unnecessary elevation of this tissue and will decrease the support surrounding the nasal bones.

Once the nasal dorsum is reduced, the septum must be reduced along its length to align with the new height of the nasal bones. The final reduction of the nasal septum is best left until after the nasal bones have been repositioned. There are times that if the dorsum of the septum is reduced prior to the final position of the nasal bones, it may again appear to be inappropriately aligned leaving either two little or too much nasal septum. If the nasal bones are reduced and positioned as a first step, then the height of the septum can be accurately ascertained preventing the need for multiple re-excisions or an over-reduced septum.

Once the nasal bones and the dorsum of the septum are aligned, the upper lateral cartilages can be trimmed in line with the height of the new septum. Care must be taken to angle the scissor in line with the septum. Over reduction of the caudal end of the lower lateral cartilage may result in that nasal valve collapse or scarring.

Once the nasal bony pyramid and septum are in alignment along with the upper lateral cartilages, it is now time to address the tip. The order of the various corrective surgical steps in any individual case is up to the surgeon. A recommended approach is to fix the tip first and then the remainder of the nose when the procedure is straightforward. This allows accurate measuring of the nasal tip structures without any additional oedema or bleeding.

Endonasal approaches to nasal tip repair

There are three endonasal techniques utilised to approach the nasal tip. These include the cartilage-splitting technique, retrograde approach, and finally the most commonly utilised, the nasal tip delivery approach. Each of these may be used depending upon the patient's individual anatomy and again the comfort level of the surgeon in carrying out the approach on the delicate nasal cartilage.

Cartilage-splitting approach

This approach is well suited for reduction of the volume of the upper alar cartilages to correct a bulbus nasal tip. It is not necessarily the method of choice for correcting existing asymmetries in the nasal tip structure. It is therefore, best utilised with symmetrical nonbifid tips that do not have a broad obtuse dome angle.

The cartilage-splitting technique allows good access to the upper alar cartilages. However, the shape of the lower alar cartilages is not altered. The intra-cartilaginous incision typically runs to the tip-defining point, which should be marked at the beginning of the case. Tip projection is unchanged when the tip defining points are preserved. This is a less invasive technique than the delivery approach and offers minimal bleeding facilitating the performance of the other endonasal operative steps.

Retrograde tip approach

The retrograde tip approach has been used since the days of the plastic surgeons who started doing cosmetic procedures following World War II. One noted surgeon was Dr Raymond Shapiro who was the first chief of plastic surgery at the Long Island Jewish Medical Center of New York. He had a personal philosophy in these early days of rhinoplasty that the fewer incisions that you do in a patient, the faster their post-operative healing time and the less chance there is for alteration of the final outcome by scar tissue formation. The instrumentation itself was not as finely developed as it is today but certainly some of his philosophy has stood the test of time.

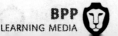

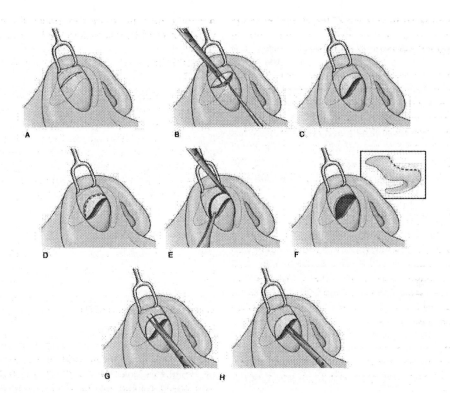

Figure 4.8: The steps in the retrograde approach

The retrograde tip approach is performed through the same intra-cartilaginous incision that is utilised to approach the dorsum of the nose. It has a limited use in that it will reduce and refine some of the bulk of the nasal tip but will not alter tip projection or height. To perform this, once the intra-cartilaginous incisions are made, a double pronged fine skin hook is now taken and the upper lateral and the cephalad end of the lower lateral cartilage is gently pulled into the nasal fossa by dissecting above the cartilage as it is retracted inferiorly with a fine iris scissor. The endonasal mucosa must also be carefully elevated off the lower lateral cartilage until a desired amount of the cephalad end of the cartilage is exposed. At this point either utilising a #15 surgical blade or the iris scissor, a section of the cartilage is removed from the cephalic leaving the caudal intact. In this way, the cartilage has maintained its position, support, and blood supply. The remaining portion of the lower lateral cartilage is allowed to merely return to its normal position. The amount of cartilage removed should be accurately measured to prevent asymmetry of the tip post-operatively.

Complete delivery approach

A complete delivery approach is an elegant endonasal technique that is recommended in the majority of cases as it gives multiple options for correcting a variety of nasal tip deformity. It does, however, require two skin incisions and elevation of a chondrocutaneous flap from the alar cartilage and the skin of the nasal vestibule. This approach requires delicacy and accuracy to not only get the desired cosmetic appearance but to prevent complications.

This procedure requires two incisions. The first is the intercartilaginous incision, which is placed in the fold between the upper lateral cartilage and the alar cartilage. This incision will be utilised to raise the skin and subcutaneous tissue over the dorsum of the nose. The skin is then incised along the caudal margin of the alar cartilage to allow the surgeon to delicately undermine the alar skin as far as the intercartilaginous incision. Care must be taken to dissect just on top of the cartilage itself to prevent disruption and scarring of the subcutaneous tissue and overlying skin with resulting unwanted deformity of the nasal tip. The alar cartilage is now delivered completely. At this point, the cartilage is in full direct view and a surgeon can make simultaneous comparisons to the size and symmetry of the cartilages. Various types of wedge resections for strips of cartilage can be performed to reduce the nasal tip volume. If the cartilage itself is too elastic and does not allow for softening of the tip outlined, the cartilage can be softened and altered with a 'tip-morseliser'. This particular type of morseliser often has the hatched surface only on one side so that you can selectively morselise one side of cartilage and not the other to control bending. Double morselisers are also available, which give an overall softening effect to the cartilage and overlying skin. This is often very useful when a patient has thin skin with little subcutaneous tissue. The surgeon may also choose to hand scroll or cross hatch the cartilage with a #15 surgical blade. Since both of the lower lateral cartilages are exposed at the same time and are in full view, resection can be measured very accurately to the millimetre and the placement of intradomal or interdomal sutures can be applied. In addition to this, if grafts need to be applied, they can be placed and sutured into position under direct vision.

How much cartilage to reduce under this particular technique has always been a matter of discussion. The traditional teachings are that a surgeon must leave 5mm of cartilage in the male nose and 4mm of cartilage in the female nose to maintain integrity and tip support while preventing the cartilage from cracking. Once cartilage is cracked or accidentally cut, the resulting edge will eventually protrude and a post-operative bocci may result giving an undesirable short tip appearance or point.

As always the surgeon must do what he or she feels comfortable with and what works best in their hands as far as how much cartilage to leave. The lower lateral cartilages must always be handled in a delicate and careful manner to disrupt the minimal amount of blood supply and to maintain post-operative support and integrity. The marginal incision is re-approximated. The intracartilaginous incision is often left open, which allows for a natural tip rotation as well as drainage, which is crucial in preventing a post-operative haematoma.

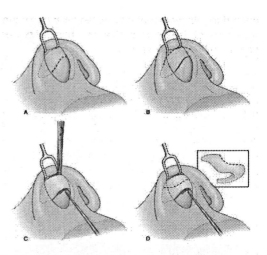

Figure 4.9 The complete delivery approach

Dome suture technique

A dome suture technique is an important part of a surgeon's set of skills and is suitable for a patient with a broad or bifid nasal tip, thin skin or subcutaneous fat and connective tissue. Interdomal sutures are used to narrow the dome. Transdomal sutures are effective for approximating the tip defining points usually after some of the intradomal fat is removed. Care must be taken in order not to pull the sutures too tightly or cut off the blood supply in the region.

There are several options for suture choice. Some authors have recommended the use of PDS for these tip suturing techniques. They felt that following suture absorption, the tip shape remains permanently stable. However, the author has found in several cases especially with weaker or ethnic type cartilage that this is not adequate and therefore uses a 4-O monofilament soft clear nylon suture to be more desirable. It is up to the individual surgeon to make these choices.

Open or decortication rhinoplasty approach

In recent years, the open approach to rhinoplasty has been popularised and has appeared more and more in our literature as well as in residency and fellowship training programmes. The advantages of

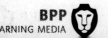

open rhinoplasty is that it provides for a maximum exposure of the alar cartilages, nasal tip and dorsum under direct vision.

The disadvantages of this technique are that it does require an external incision, which can always result in scar tissue formation and a somewhat delayed healing time. However, when the nasal structure requires such visualisation, often with the placement of additional grafts or the increased comfort of the surgeon in performing this particular nasal procedure, it is a very important part of the armamentarium that helps the patient to obtain an excellent cosmetic result.

Procedure

A skin incision is made in a W-configuration or often referred to as a stepped zigzagged incision at the mid-columellar level. The incision is then carefully carried around the medial crura extending on to the lateral columella and then joins with the marginal alar incisions. The skin is undermined with fine iris scissors or appropriate scissors. The columellar flap is progressively developed and extended superiorly. When the medial crura of the alar cartilages have been exposed, the medial surface provides a guide for dissecting in the cephalad direction. A dissection is then carried on top of the alar dome and then laterally over the lower lateral cartilages. From here the dissection can be carried over the upper lateral cartilages on to the nasal bone with complete elevation of the nasal dorsum skin and soft and connective tissue. At the end of the dissection, the lower lateral cartilages, the upper lateral cartilages, the valve region, and nasal bones up to the frontomaxillary process can be seen. Some authors indicate a supraperichondrial dissection and then a subperiosteal plain at the level of the rhinion.

The advantages of this approach include a binocular, three-dimensional view with the ability to dissect the structures bimanually with good haemostatic control. Additionally, accurate resection of the different areas of both cartilage and bone can be conducted to achieve symmetry especially in a patient who has pre-operative nasal asymmetry. The placement of various types of grafts both large and small can be accurately

positioned and sutured in place to prevent post-operative displacement. The different types of grafts can be held in place with a suture of the surgeon's choice. Most commonly 5-O PDS as well as 4-O clear mono soft nylon.

Once the nasal structures have been reduced or trimmed to the desired amount and haemostasis is assured the skin and dorsum of the nose as well as columellar flap can be returned to its original position. Accurate realignment of the columellar incision must be achieved to prevent scar tissue formation. The columella can be sutured with a 6-O nylon suture. The intranasal portion of the incisions can be closed with a 4-O chromic absorbable suture. A nasal splint and packing as necessitated by the procedure are placed in a normal fashion.

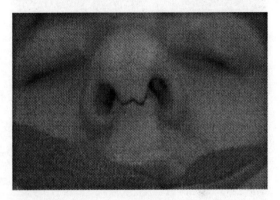

Figure 4.10 Columella incision

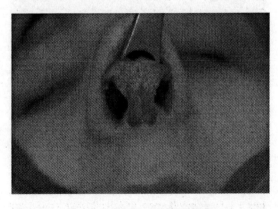

Figure 4.11 Exposed lower lateral cartilage

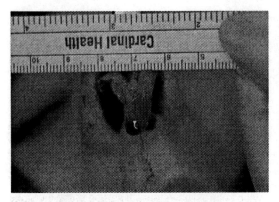

Figure 4.12 Trimming lower lateral cartilage

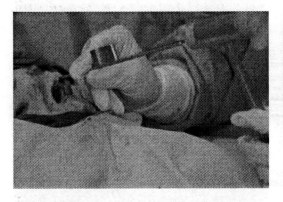

Figure 4.13 Reducing the dorsal nasal hump

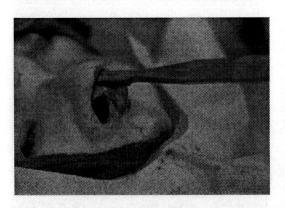

Figure 4.14 Rasping the nasal dorsum

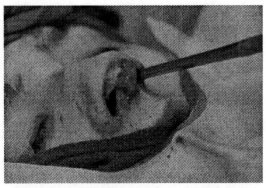

Figure 4.15 Lateral osteotomy

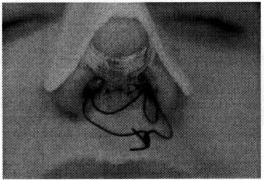

Figure 4.16 Post-operative packing and splint

Nasal grafts

The use of as few nasal grafts as possible by being careful not to over resect either the bone or nasal cartilage structures should always be the goal. However, there are times when the patient's particular nasal structure does necessitate the use of a graft to correct a prior deformity or enhance the desired cosmetic result. One important point must be made at this time in choosing grafting material, it is better to avoid the use of any form of artificial grafting material in the nose such as silicone or Gore-Tex®. Although some of this material may be appropriate for other areas in facial contouring such as cheeks, chin, or lips, it is not suitable for the nose. The paucity of subcutaneous tissue underneath the nasal skin makes this a dangerous place to put anything but an autologous graft. Some of the artificial grafting material may look good for a while, sometimes a minor amount of nasal trauma will set a cascade in motion resulting in this artificial grafting material being rejected, often directly through the nasal skin with a disastrous outcome. Most of these unfortunate mishaps can be avoided by choosing an appropriate autologous graft material from cartilage or bone harvested from the excess nasal structures themselves, conchal ear cartilage or, for major reconstructions, rib bone and/or cartilage.

Columella strut

This is one of the most widely utilised nasal grafts and can be made up in either cartilage and/or bone harvested from the nose. It is placed in a pocket between the basal medial crura of the alar cartilages over the anterior nasal spine and fixed between the medial crura with through and through sutures. This graft is commonly used to control tip projection and provides tip support especially in the nose which is under projected. It is commonly used in the ethnic nose.

Onlay grafts

Onlay grafts are used on the nasal dorsum or lateral alar cartilages to correct for the loss of substance or to contour the nose. This is a very common graft utilised in a secondary or revision rhinoplasty procedure. Again, this should be approached with all precautions about the placement of artificial grafting material in this area because of the risk of eventual loss of the material by extrusion through the skin even from a minor nasal trauma months or even years after placement.

Spreader grafts

The spreader graft has been reserved for last since it again is one of the most commonly used in primary and secondary rhinoplasty. The graft is placed extra-mucosally between the dorsal septum and the upper lateral cartilages. It is utilised both for function and for cosmetic effects. The graft is often placed after the removal of a large hump or in a large nose with short nasal bones. The spreader grafts have been utilised to prevent post-operative nasal valve stenosis and to create a harmonious eye brow-tip line.

Placement of grafting material in this region has also been utilised to help prevent re-deviation of a nasal septum which has been corrected.

End results

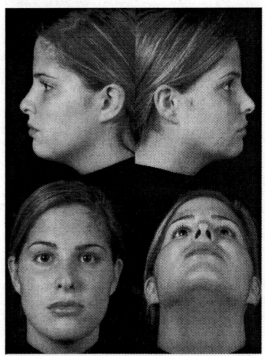

Figure 4.17 Post-operative rhinoplasty views

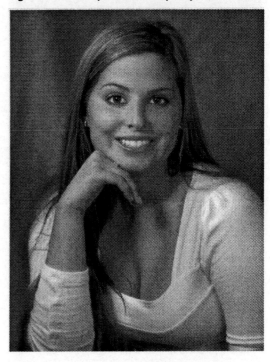

Figure 4.18: Post-operative rhinoplasty frontal view

Blepharoplasty

Blepharoplasty is the alteration of the soft tissue around the eye and eyelids, which results in the restoration of a more youthful appearance of the periorbital area and a less fatigued or tired look. It is often said that the eyes are the windows to the soul and represent one of the most expressive and emotional features of the human face. This is the reason that any error in technique or results in this region are immediately magnified. However a good cosmetic result in this region may dramatically affect one's appearance more than almost any other facial cosmetic surgery.

The orbicularis oculi muscle is located directly beneath the skin of the eyelid and is divided into the palpebral and orbital portions. The palpebral portion is further subdivided into pretarsal and preseptal muscles. The preseptal muscle contracts in a circular pattern thus elevating the lower lid.

The tarsal plate of both the upper and lower eyelids is composed of a dense fibrous connective tissue. The tarsal plates support the eyelids and attach to the medial and lateral canthal ligaments. The upper tarsus is supported primarily by the levator palpebrae superioris muscle. The lower tarsus is supported by the orbital septum. This orbital septum is an extension of the lower tarsus and is joined by the fascia from the inferior oblique muscle. Additional support comes from the inferior aponeurosis of the capsulopalpebral head of the inferior rectus muscle, which corresponds to the levator muscle of the upper lid.

The periorbital adipose tissue is contained in five separate compartments in each eye. Two compartments are in the upper lid and three in the lower lid. There are several theories about the aetiology of the adipose tissue in the eye: one states that it is mostly hereditary and not related to the patient's body weight.

The orbital fat is mostly visible in the medial compartment of the upper eyelid and the three lower eyelid compartments – medial, central, and, less frequently, lateral. The areas of protruding orbital fat are frequently called herniated fat pads, although this may not be technically correct. In reality the apparent protrusion of this orbital adipose tissue is caused by relaxation or weakness of the orbital septum. All the patients may however have some actual herniation.

Anatomy

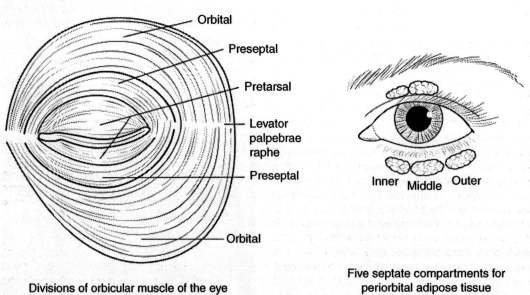

Divisions of orbicular muscle of the eye

Five septate compartments for periorbital adipose tissue

Figure 4.19 Orbicularis occuli muscle and peri-orbital fat compartments

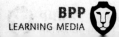

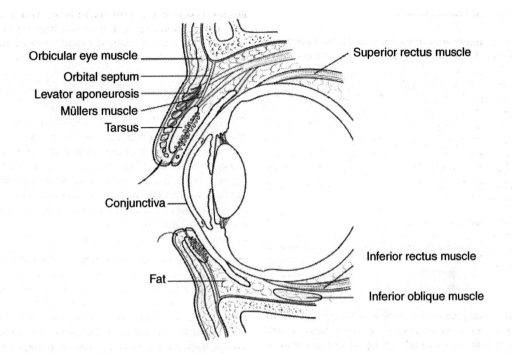

Figure 4.20: Cross section of orbit and eyelids

The cosmetic surgeon must always take in to consideration anatomy and a possibility of normal structures presenting themselves during surgery with a risk of injury. This is sometime seen where the inferior oblique muscle runs between the medial and central fat pads of the lower lid. Here it is extremely susceptible to injury during dissection.

Another anatomical structure that may be easily injured during blepharoplasty is the lacrimal gland. It is estimated that 15% of patients who undergo blepharoplasty exhibit a displacement of the lacrimal gland and therefore may be more susceptible to injury of the structure. If the displacement of the lacrimal gland is not corrected during surgery, then the post-operative result may show continued fullness in the lateral aspect of the lid. The lacrimal gland itself is pink in colour, is in the superior temporal quadrant of the orbit and is separated from the fat compartments by the lateral horn of the levator aponeurosis. It therefore does not resemble orbital adipose tissue. The presence of fullness in the lateral aspect of the upper eyelid should at once raise suspicion of displacement of the lacrimal gland. This finding is more common in females than males.

Classification of eyelid deformities

There are several different deformities of the upper and lower eyelids. There are six such deformities which fall into the realm of cosmetic blepharoplasty.

1. Blepharochalasis

2. Dermatochalasis

3. Hypertrophy of the orbicularis muscle

4. Protrusion of intraorbital fat

5. Combination of these conditions

6. Hooding of the upper lids because of ptosis of the eyebrows

1. **Blepharochalasis** is defined as atony or relaxation at the lid skin that becomes wrinkled and hangs like a curtain over the eyes. This is of undetermined aetiology.

2. **Dermatochalasis** is also categorised by some surgeons as ptosis adiposa of Sichel, but this is in fact a misnomer since there is no subcutaneous adipose tissue in the eye lid. This condition involves primarily the upper lids and is essentially hypertrophy of the upper eyelid skin. In dermatochalasis,

the fascial bands that connect the skin with the orbicularis muscle and the orbital ostium become relaxed allowing the thickened and relaxed skin to hang down over the eyes.

3. **Hypertrophy of the orbicularis muscle** is different, but can coexist with 1 and 2 (above). This condition is commonly found in individuals who are constantly squinting or smiling. The deformity appears immediately below the lower lid margin. This bulging is different than that which is caused by the protrusion of orbital fat. Hypertrophy of the orbicularis muscle is most commonly treated by a wedge resection of the muscle tissue.

4. **Protrusion (herniation) of intraorbital fat** is a major cause of eyelid deformities. The condition can be found in young as well as older patients and has no sexual predilection. This is thought to be hereditary in nature. Protrusion of the orbital fat occurs because of weakness in the tarsal orbital septum and orbicularis muscle. It therefore is not a herniation in the true sense of the word as there is no actual break in the fascia or muscle.

5. A **combination of these conditions** can be seen and coexist in the same patient.

6. **Hooding of the upper eyelids** occurs in many individuals. This lid deformity is secondary to descent of the eyebrows in a general ageing process of the face. This condition must be recognised so that surgical correction can be aimed at the proper anatomical region, which is the eyebrows and not the eyelids.

Patient selection

Blepharoplasty is performed commonly for two specific reasons:

1. Excess skin of eyelids

2. Protrusion of orbital fat often caused by relaxation of the orbital septum

A properly performed blepharoplasty can be one of the most satisfying cosmetic procedures. However, if it is not performed properly, it can result in truly significant disfigurement. A pre-operative evaluation is therefore essential. As with many cosmetic procedures psychological evaluation and

preparation of the patient is at the top of the list. The patient must have a realistic understanding of what they hope to accomplish with this surgery and what will not be achieved with the surgery.

As with any other patient, a good medical history is a prime importance. A surgeon must be aware of disorders that can affect the surgical outcome including thyroid diseases, chronic renal disorders, coagulopathies, especially patients who are on anticoagulant therapy including aspirin or Plavix etc, cardiac conditions, chronic steroid therapy, blinking spasms, and ticks or other ophthalmological conditions. A personal or family history of glaucoma, past orbital trauma, recurrent ophthalmic infections or other problems such as dry eyes should be ascertained.

Physical examination of the orbit and facial areas should be part of any pre-operative examination for blepharoplasty. Mild pressure on the globes may delineate the prominent fat pads. If wrinkles lateral to the eyes are noted, the patient should be told that this will not be improved by the blepharoplasty. This is frequently a small but very important point in the post-operative satisfaction of the patient. Increased pigmentation of the periorbital skin should also be noted and the patient is informed that this may not be eliminated by this type of surgery and indeed may in fact be increased.

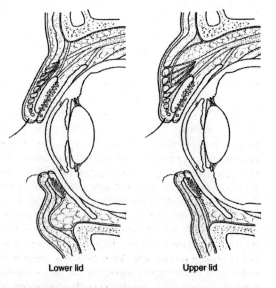

Lower lid   Upper lid

Figure 4.21 Cross section of orbit and eyelids showing protrusion of peri-orbital fat into lower and upper eyelids respectively

Photographic documentation is important. Six different views are often taken for complete evaluation.

Many surgeons feel strongly that each patient should get a presurgical ophthalmological evaluation. Many times, this examination will uncover underlying problems that may actually be a contraindication to this type of surgery. The ophthalmologist will perform the usual examination but it is very important that the patient undergo Schirmer's test to evaluate the possibility of a dry eye post-operatively, which can be a very difficult problem to treat. If the patient has significant visual field loss, this should of course be noted especially in the superior fields as many patients undergo blepharoplasty to improve their visual field loss. A letter documenting the ophthalmologic examination should be obtained and placed in the patient's chart.

Procedure

Anaesthesia

Blepharoplasty can be performed using local or general anaesthesia. When blepharoplasty is being performed as the only procedure it may be preferable to do this under local anaesthesia with some intravenous sedation. When performed under local anaesthetic, the patient can respond to commands to test extraocular movements at various times during the procedure, which may allow the surgeon to adjust the amount of tissue to excise. Local anaesthetic can reduce bruising or swelling and the patient can protect their eyes when excessive pulling or tugging on ocular structures exist or when the patient is starting to get corneal irritation.

However, usually the blepharoplasty is being performed as part of a larger procedure or patients do not care to be awake. Properly performed general anaesthesia, combined with the use of local anaesthetic and haemostatic agents, remains a safe procedure. Regardless of which type of anaesthesia is used, a key part of the process is to be sure to have absolute and meticulous haemostasis. This is more important in blepharoplasty than almost any other cosmetic procedure, haemostasis is crucial in preventing a significant post-operative complication. After injecting a local anaesthetic agent eg 1:200

lidocaine (lignocaine) with 1/100,000 epinephrine (adrenaline), light pressure is applied to reduce bruising at the surgical site. Approximately 20 minutes of time is allowed for the local anaesthetic agent to reach its full effect before starting any surgical procedure.

Surgical technique: points of consideration

There are several points which the cosmetic surgeon performing blepharoplasty should be aware of.

1. When the surgeon is dissecting the medial portion of the upper lid, they should not extend the incision into the lateral nasal skin. This could result in a bridle scar and is generally unattractive and deforming. If redundant tissue was noted in this region then it should be removed in a standard dog-ear fashion. The burrow's triangle is excised and closed in a standard fashion, which will result in a cosmetically pleasing appearance.

2. The lateral portion of the lower eyelid incision should not extend above the lateral canthal region. You should leave at least 4mm of tissue between the lateral portion of the upper and lower lid incisions. This is important to allow adequate vascular drainage.

3. The upper eyelid blepharoplasty should be performed first and the lateral portion of the lid incision sutured close. This increased elevation of the upper eyelid closure may affect the amount of lower eyelid skin that should be removed thereby preventing a post-operative problem or complication.

4. The lower lid incision should not extend medial to the lower lacrimal punctum as this may cause a disruption of the lacrimal apparatus.

5. There are two basic surgical techniques for the lower lid blepharoplasty. One is a skin flap only and the second is a skin and muscle flap. The skin-muscle flap technique is advocated in the majority of blepharoplasties for several reasons. Most commonly the redundant tissue that is causing the sagging lower lid is composed

of both skin and the attached orbicularis oculi muscle. To correct the deformity you must address both the skin and muscle. In addition to this, the anatomic plane between the muscle and the orbital septum is easily dissected and relatively avascular. This surgery should be performed with a minimal amount of soft tissue trauma. In addition, the skin muscle flap allows a more complete exposure of the orbital septum and permits better visualisation and excision with increased haemostatic control of the protruding orbital fat.

6.   A strip of orbicularis muscle is often removed from the lower lid skin flap to create a more pleasing contour to the lower lid. This can be accomplished by bevelling the scissors in an inferior direction when making the final cuts along the lower eyelid thereby resecting more muscle than skin.

7.   Immediate application of ice saline compresses significantly reduces the postsurgical oedema and ecchymosis. It is good practice to start the ice saline compresses in the operating room initially on the first eye while operating on the second eye.

Post-operative instructions

A written sheet of post-operative instructions is supplied to all patients. Most surgeons find that despite talking to both patients and family pre-operatively, as with many other pre-operative discussions, some of this is soon forgotten and a written sheet handed to the patient and family is much more effective.

Post-operative instructions:

1.   Sleep with the head elevated on at least two pillows for approximately one week.

2.   Apply ice compresses every 20 minutes following the surgery. Continue ice compresses for two days after surgery, applying them for 20 minutes every two hours.

3.   Clean incision lines with a sterile cotton swab and peroxide three times a day, being careful not to get it into the eyes.

4.   Apply a bead of ophthalmic bacitracin ointment to the suture lines, twice a day.

5.   Take only prescribed pain medication or paracetamol/acetaminophen if advised. Do not take aspirin or ibuprofen containing products.

6.   Shower on the second or third day after surgery being careful not to allow any force of the water to go directly on to the suture lines.

7.   Report any excessive pain, bleeding or changes in vision immediately to your doctor or go to the nearest emergency room.

Post-operative complications of blepharoplasty and management

Haematoma

The best post-operative treatment for haematoma is prevention by meticulous haemostasis at the time of surgery. If a haematoma is noted in the immediate post-operative, evacuation should be performed as soon as possible. Following this, additional mild pressure and cold compresses should be utilised to prevent its recurrence. If a haematoma is noted several days following the procedure, some authors advocate allowing it to liquefy and aspirate with a 10ml syringe and #18-gauge needle. Haematoma formation occurs in approximately 3% of blepharoplasties. The most significant problem from the haematoma is spreading of blood and increased ocular pressure with loss of vision. It is for this reason that haemostasis is crucial.

Oedema

Oedema occurs in almost all blepharoplasty patients to a variable degree. It is more of a known occurrence than a complication of the surgery. It usually will clear spontaneously causing no significant problem. It can always be lessened by the use of cold compresses post-operatively and elevation of the patient's bed.

Ulcers of the cornea

Corneal ulceration was more commonly seen when utilising either too strong an electric current

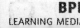

when coagulating bleeding sites or with monopolar cautery. Thermal injuries to orbital tissue can occur even with lower disposable battery powered cautery. The sensitivity of orbital tissue to thermal injury is variable. The lacrimal gland tissue appears to be more sensitive than fat and muscle. The known complications from cauterisation include corneal ulceration and extraocular muscle paresis. If there is significant fat necrosis, an intense inflammatory reaction may be noted post-operatively with the potential for marked fibrosis. It is for these reasons that bipolar coagulation is the method of choice. In today's modern era, unless you are operating in a field hospital, there is no reason why the modern cosmetic surgeon would not have a bipolar cautery present.

The advantages of bipolar current include minimal current spread to the adjacent tissue, a minimal amount of current is necessary to obtain the desired haemostatic result, elimination of undesired secondary burns and effective coagulation even when irrigation is present. The essential advantage in bipolar coagulation is the absence of an electrical contact with the patient and a concentration of current flow through uninvolved tissues. Because the current is limited to the region of the tip of the forceps only, the surgeon must be very accurate in his/her application. This should not however be considered a disadvantage.

Cysts

Small retention cysts of sebaceous glands can occur frequently in the upper eyelid following blepharoplasty and to a lesser extent in the lower eyelid. This particular complication can be reduced by the utilisation of a continuous subcuticular stitch as opposed to an over and over technique, where suture material is seen to extend outside of the skin.

Wound separation

Wound separation occurs for various reasons and is most commonly seen when the patient inadvertently rubs their incision resulting in a mild wound dehiscence. This can be treated by either re-suturing the incision or applying Steri-Strips. Many patients are advised to wear dark glasses not only to protect their eyes from the sunlight but also to remind them not to rub the eyes and the surgical incision site.

Scars

This is a more of a problem in darkly pigmented individuals who may become depigmented several months after surgery. The assurance that coloration problems will resolve is the only treatment needed at this time.

Ectropion

Ectropion refers to the loss of the normally close approximation of the margin of the lid with the underlying globe of the eye. Loss of this approximation leads not only to an unsightly cosmetic defect but incompetence of lid function. The latter is one of the most frequent and serious blepharoplasty complications, more commonly associated with lower lid blepharoplasty. Ectropion of the upper eyelid is rare, presumably because of the larger tarsal plate.

Several factors may account for the development of an ectropion. The orbital septum is somewhat inelastic and if a surgeon re-sutures the septum, it may shorten the vertical height. Resuturing of the orbital septum is usually not necessary as long as sufficient orbital fat has been removed. Many surgeons feel the single most important causative factor in ectropion of the lower eyelid is excessive removal of skin from the lower eyelid at surgery. This error may occur in part because the patient is lying recumbent on the operating room table. The full gravitational effect on the cheeks and lower face may be underestimated especially when the surgery is being performed under a general anaesthetic. Therefore, always erring on the side of conservative resection will help in reducing the chance of this complication. If the patient is awake, the surgeon may ask them to look superiorly and open their mouth as wide as possible. This will allow the surgeon to evaluate and compensate for the pull of gravity.

Another common cause of ectropion in the older patient is the lack of tone of the lateral canthal tendon, called an atonic lower lid. This condition can be noticed pre-operatively by seeing if the patient has a good 'snap test'. The snap test is performed by gently grasping the lower eye lid and pulling it away from the eye. It is then released and the surgeon can see how quickly it returns or snaps back to its original position. This will help indicate pre-operatively whether the canthal tendon has adequate support. A lateral canthal

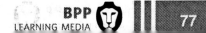

tendon suspension suture at the time of surgery can be used to improve the tone of the tendon.

Many patients have a transient period of ectropion of several days to a week following blepharoplasty during which the lateral half of the lower eyelid assumes an abnormally low position. This is usually secondary to oedema of the skin and conjunctiva and generally resolves spontaneously.

Frequently, conservative treatment will correct the milder forms of ectropion over a period of several weeks, by forceful squinting, massaging in a superolateral direction and applying Steri-Strips. Massage should be performed for 10 to 15 minutes four to five times a day. At night, the patient should place tape at the lateral lid margin to help support the eyelid in a more superolateral direction. If the patient starts to exhibit symptoms of a dry eye, then liquid tears and/or ophthalmic lubricating ointment must be prescribed to help prevent corneal ulceration.

If severe ectropion is noted in the immediate post-operative period while the patient is still in the operating room, it is mostly caused by excessive resection of the lower eyelid skin and correction may be undertaken immediately. The skin excised from the upper eyelid can be placed as a skin graft that will eliminate the lower lid ectropion.

The excised upper eyelid skin can be stored gauze soaked in normal saline at 40 degrees centigrade for use within 24 to 48 hours post-operatively in case a severe ectropion were to develop. . A tie-over dressing should be placed for approximately 7 to 10 days. The final appearance may be quite satisfying. If this opportunity to utilise the skin in the immediate post-operative period is missed, it is better to delay grafting for several months. New skin may be obtained from the postauricular region with a good colour match.

Dry eyes (keratoconjunctivitis sicca)

It is not uncommon for a patient to experience some increased tearing or epiphora following blepharoplasty even if uncomplicated. This is generally secondary to oedema and is transitory. However, if the tearing remains excessive it may be caused by irritative reflex hypersecretion, a symptom of inadequate tear production. In these patients dry eyes should be suspected, especially in the older patient. If dry eyes are noted post-operatively, the patient should be given liquid tears and followed by an ophthalmologist. Often the condition is transient, however, some patients may need to continue on artificial tears for a significant period of time.

Blindness

Blindness is probably the most dreaded complication of blepharoplasty. This has been reported by some authors to occur in one in 25,000 patients. Blindness following blepharoplasty has been attributed to multiple causes including optic neuritis, multiple sclerosis, brain aneurysm, glaucoma, orbital cellulitis and infraorbital haemorrhage.

If orbital cellulitis occurs, immediate hospitalisation and intravenous antibiotic therapy are recommended.

Infraorbital haemorrhage can occur as a complication of blepharoplasty and is felt to be secondary to traction on orbital fat during dissection. This results in tearing of the penetrating branches of the infraorbital vessels that run from the main trunks, fixed in the bony grooves of the orbital floor. In addition, bleeding from transected vessels in the pedicle of the fat pads is a likely cause. Bleeding has been known to occur as a result of post-operative vomiting and/or straining following administration of anaesthetics or other drugs, which may make the patient nauseous.

As a cosmetic surgeon performing blepharoplasty, it is important to have a complete understanding of intraocular pressure. The average pressure in the aqueous and vitreous of the human eye is 15.5mmHg. The vitreous compartment of the eye is relatively static and does not produce fluctuations in intraocular pressure. The aqueous compartment is dynamic and forms fluid at the rate of 4 micro litres per minute by the ciliary process of the eye. The total volume of both chambers is approximately 0.4ml. Aqueous is produced continuously. For this reason, it must be eliminated at a continuous rate or there will be an increase in intraocular pressure. Normally pressure within the ocular system remains constant. However, if there is a sudden increase, the iris may be pushed forward to occlude Schlemm's canal. This may result in an acute increase in intraocular pressure above the normal 15.5mmHg.

A retrobulbar haemorrhage results in dissection of the bleeding intraorbital fat, muscles, and other structures. This can increase intraorbital pressure.

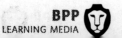

The pressure will continue to rise until it reaches the level of the systolic blood pressure. At this point, the bleeding will subside but it will also decrease blood flow to the central retinal artery thus resulting in blindness.

The retina is extremely sensitive to diminished oxygen tension: approximately six minutes of diminished blood flow result in permanent retinal damage and possibly total blindness. For this reason, the cosmetic surgeon must be able to identify the problem and react quickly to prevent any serious side effects secondary to the retrobulbar haematoma. Any surgeon performing blepharoplasty should have available an emergency eye tray that includes instruments for decompressing the wound under local anaesthesia as well as medication such as 20% mannitol.

Should an acute visual loss occur secondary to what is believed to be a retrobulbar haematoma the following steps should be taken immediately.

1.   All wounds should be opened including violated orbital septum.

2.   If the patient continues to have increased intraocular pressure, a lateral canthotomy should be performed.

3.   If increased ocular pressure continues, attempts should be made to lower the intraocular pressure by use of a hyperosmotic agent such as intravenous mannitol or acetazolamide. 12.5g mannitol should be given intravenously within a period of three to five minutes and then followed with slow administration so that total dose will be 1 to 2g of mannitol per kilogram of the patient's body weight within the next 30 minutes. If loss of vision persists for ten minutes, an ophthalmologist must perform an anterior chamber paracentesis. During this surgery, a thin cataract knife can be introduced into the anterior chamber through the limbus parallel to the iris and anterior to Schlemm's canal. This results in immediate outflow of the aqueous fluid. After 0.3 to 0.4ml of aqueous fluid has been evacuated, the pressure will be reduced in the anterior chamber and the iris can move in to its normal position and allow normal aqueous flow through via Schlemm's canal. The aqueous volume regenerates very quickly in approximately ten minutes.

As retrobulbar haematoma has potentially serious and permanent effects resulting in blindness, as soon as this may be suspected an experienced ophthalmologist should be consulted immediately. The previous steps should be performed, pending the arrival of the ophthalmologist. However, only an experienced individual should perform the anterior chamber paracentesis.

Rhytidectomy

Rhytidectomy is the technical term for what is commonly known as a face-lift. There have been many surgical and technical variations to attempt to gain the most cosmetic pleasing result with maximal patient satisfaction and least amount of complications. Ultimately, we will see that which particular procedure is utilised depends upon patient selection as well as the surgeon's own technical skill and surgical beliefs. As in all other surgical procedures, patient selection is the first, and often most important, factor in a successful outcome.

It is often felt that the ideal rhytidectomy candidate would be a thin, fair-skinned, middle aged female, in good health with a minimal amount of subcutaneous adipose tissue and a maximal amount of skin laxity of jowl line and neck. Conversely a stocky overweight individual with thick hyperpigmented skin may obtain less than optimal results. The overall aim of rhytidectomy is to obtain a smooth contour and tightening of the jowl line, elevate sagging cheeks, improve facial expression lines from the downward position to the more youthful superior and posterior orientation, reduce the prominence of the buccolabial folds and finally to reduce the redundancy and bulkiness in the submental and cervical region. Ultimately, it is the patient selection and not just the surgical technique which will allow some if not all of these ideals to be achieved.

Facial anatomy

As in all other surgical procedures a thorough understanding of the regional anatomy is a paramount importance. This is crucial in obtaining not only the desired result but decreasing the chance for untoward side effects.

Facial muscular anatomy

The facial muscles are divided into five groups; oral, nasal, orbital and muscles of the ear and scalp. The platysma muscle in the neck also belongs to this facial group. The lower group of oral muscles which are innervated primarily through the marginal mandibular nerve, a branch of the facial nerve, consists of depressor anguli, depressor labii inferioris, and mentalis. The upper group of oral muscles includes the risorius, the main innervation of which is via the buccal branch of the facial nerve; the zygomaticus (major and minor) main innervation via the upper buccal and zygomatic branches of the facial nerve; the levators, orbicularis oris, and buccinator muscles. The nasal group of muscles includes the nasalis, depressor septi and dilator muscles. The orbicularis oculi, procerus, and corrugator supercilii make up the orbital muscle group. The fifth group of cervicofacial muscles, the muscles of the ear and scalp, consists of the extrinsic muscles of the ear and epicranial muscles.

Superficial musculoaponeurotic system (SMAS)

In 1976, Mitz and Peyronie (1976) noted that a cutaneous fascial layer exists and extends from the superficial surface of the frontalis muscle in conjunction with the superficial temporal fascia, inferiorly over the zygoma, buccal region and parotid gland, and superficial surface of the platysma. They noted that the fascia was associated with the muscles of the face and was connected vertically to the more superficial dermis. No significant vascularity had been noted. In addition to this, no motor nerves were located superficial to the SMAS in the layer of routine rhytidectomy dissection.

The modality of the rhytidectomy using the concepts of limited undermining and fascial plication supports cutaneous facial structures by advancing and repositioning the underlying fascia or SMAS. This particular technique has been utilised with success for many years. In the classic long flap rhytidectomy some surgeons felt that the extensive undermining would weaken some of the connections between the SMAS and the dermis thereby decreasing the desired suspension effects of tightening the SMAS.

Blood supply

The external carotid artery supplies most of the fascial tissue through branches of the facial or external maxillary arteries.

Veins

Drainage for the facial tissue is chiefly through the facial vein. The angular vein has free communication with the ophthalmic vein. There is also communication with the veins to the forehead, lips, nose and orbital region. The facial vein transverses the surface of the submandibular gland en route to the internal jugular vein.

Of importance to note is that the absence of valves in the facial veins results in a free communication with the facial and ophthalmic veins. Since the ophthalmic vein connects with the cavernous sinus, any infection of the facial tissues can easily spread intracranially. Prophylactic antibiotics may be considered when performing rhytidectomy.

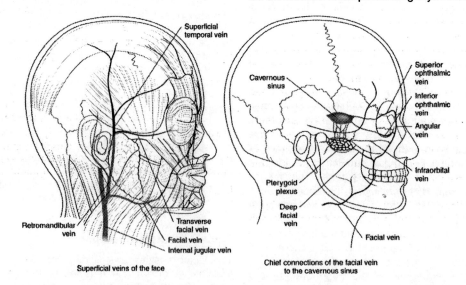

Superficial veins of the face

Chief connections of the facial vein to the cavernous sinus

Figure 4.22: Anatomy of superficial facial veins and their deep connections

Nervous system

Motor nerves

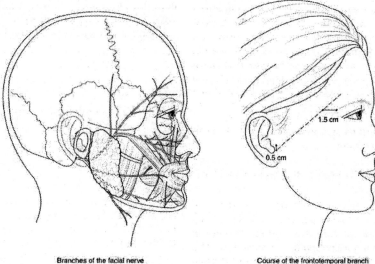

Branches of the facial nerve

Course of the frontotemporal branch of the facial nerve

Figure 4.23 Branches of the facial nerve

The facial nerve is the primary motor nerve to the muscles. The seventh cranial nerve is divided into five branches including temporal zygomatic buccal, marginal mandibular, and cervical. Paralysis of either the buccal or marginal mandibular nerve or both produces the greatest facial deformity. These nerves are responsible for innervating the highly mobile perioral region. The anatomy of these facial nerves frequently varies. The frontotemporal branch is the most variable in its course and therefore the most at risk of injury during rhytidectomy. This nerve innervates the superior one-third of the face and has a constant direction. The course of this nerve may be represented by a line starting 0.5cm inferior to the tragus and extending to a point 1.5cm above the lateral aspect of the eyebrow.

This guideline is extremely useful in identifying the course of the nerve during rhytidectomy. The marginal mandibular nerve commonly follows a course below the angle of the mandible that arcs anteriorly and superiorly toward the perioral musculature. This nerve is often located in the region of the facial artery and vein. Facelift dissection in this area can therefore damage this nerve branch.

Sensory nerves

The sensory nerves supply to the face is primarily via the trigeminal or fifth cranial nerve. The cervical plexus (C2, C3 and a portion of C4) supplies the inferior portion of the mandible. Cranial nerves VII, IX and X supply the greater portion of the external auricle. Most of the other facial structures are innervated by the trigeminal nerve.

Variations and surgical techniques for rhytidectomy

Long versus short flap

Over the years, there has been much controversy about which approach provides the most satisfactory long-term cosmetic results. Surgeons who believe in limited or conservative undermining are just as many as those who believe that more extensive undermining is better. Many studies and reports have been undertaken comparing limited versus extensive undermining.

Extensive undermining was defined as that which is carried to the lateral canthus, malar prominence, and to the buccolabial fold, mental foramen, and into the neck to the level of the thyroid cartilage. Limited undermining is defined as dissection to one half of the distance from the incision to the reference points. The anterior margin of the limited undermining flap can be measured starting at the tragus and moving anteriorly on the face 4cm. The other key points of the undermining can be seen in Figure 4.24. Studies have demonstrated that even with extensive undermining only 15% more skin as compared to limited undermining could be resected. There was little discernible difference between the static results obtained by other

procedures. A SMAS plication was employed in all cases. However, 80% of complications occurred on the extensively undermined procedures. In addition to reducing the risk of complication, there appears to be less impairment of circulation and more tension could safely be applied to the short flaps. It was also noted that more rapid healing was obtained in the less undermined flaps.

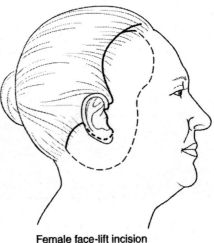

Female face-lift incision

Figure 4.25 Female face-lift incision

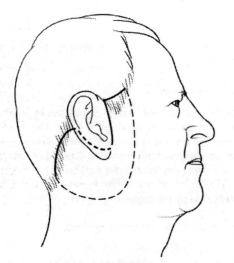

Male face-lift incision

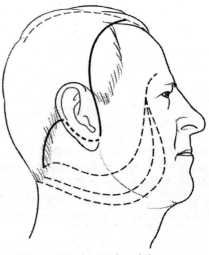

More extensive undermining

Figure 4.24: Male face-lift incision showing limited and more extensive undermining

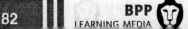

Plication and imbrication of SMAS

Over the years, many surgeons have utilised techniques that employ plication or imbrication of the fascial tissue plains. Plication is defined as suturing the folds of the fascial layer on itself while imbrication, by cutting the excess tissue and then suturing in place, may result in a flatter edge of tissue to overlap the deep structures. Regardless of which technique is utilised, imbricating or plicating the SMAS layer improves the long lasting effects especially in the neck and jowl region. SMAS plication is only an adjunct to the procedure and is not a substitute for adequate proper skin or adipose tissue resection.

Surgical procedure

Regardless of the anterior incision, the post auricular incision is carried into the hairline at approximately the level of an imaginary line drawn through the external auditory canal. The hairline incision is carried for a distance of approximately 3 to 4cm, it is angular inferiorly to eliminate any tissue redundancy or dog-ear. New hair growths will often camouflage any incision lines in this region. Incisions in the hair bearing area are bevelled in the direction parallel to the direction of the growth of the hair follicles to avoid hair loss or alopecia.

The temple incision follows a gentle curve of the hairline approximately 1 to 2cm in the hair bearing area. In this way, the scar will again be hidden with new hair growth. The temple incision may be carried as far superiorly and medially as necessary to eliminate laxity of the forehead skin and provide adequate support to the eyebrows. It is not uncommon that these incisions are extended to meet bilaterally and a coronal forehead lift may be developed as necessary.

In the male facelift patient, the incisions are often modified. The temporal incision may be limited to prevent an unsightly scar should male pattern baldness develop later in life. A preauricular incision in males is preferable.

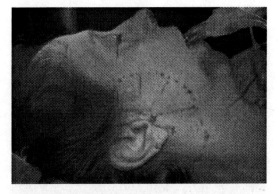

Figure 4.26 Making the site of incisions and undermining right side of face

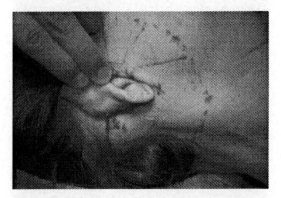

Figure 4.27 Site of post-auricular rhytidectomy incision

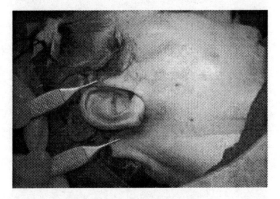

Figure 4.28 Rhytidectomy flap elevated

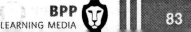

End results

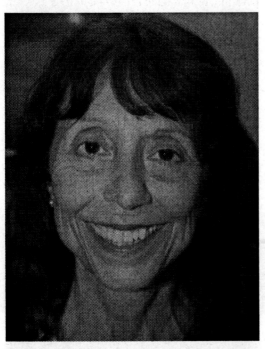

Figure 4.29 Rhytidectomy pre-operative frontal view

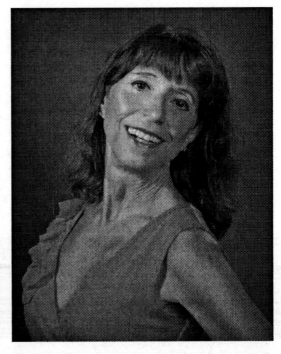

Figure 4.31 Rhytidectomy post-operative oblique view

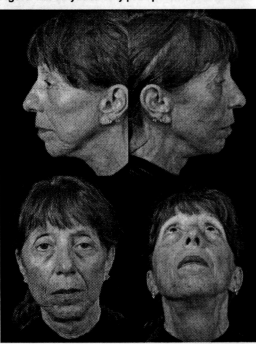

Figure 4.30 Rhytidectomy pre-operative additional views

Complications of rhytidectomy

Haematoma formation is one of the most frequent complications of rhytidectomy and is estimated to occur in up to 15% of patients. To a much lesser extent, it would be considered significant enough to require surgical intervention. As with many other surgical procedures, the best treatment for haematoma is to avoid one during the procedure itself. The use of meticulous haemostasis, bipolar cautery, and a well positioned surgical dressing, will all help in avoiding haematoma formation. If a haematoma does develop, it can be removed with minimal intervention utilising a 10ml syringe and #18 gauge needle. If not, a few sutures or staples can be removed and the haematoma milked out through the incision line. Major haematoma formation requires surgical intervention to protect skin flap viability. Pain is the most common and frequent complaint of a patient who is developing a haematoma. As with many other cosmetic procedures, post-operative nausea and vomiting are linked to haematoma formation. Coughing is also a problem in this entity and it may be important to use antipertussants post-operatively, if it develops. Careful attention must be placed on the pre-operative evaluation and history of any medicine or vitamin intake. Anticoagulants and vitamins which prolong bleeding times must be stopped a minimum of two weeks prior to surgery.

Necrosis of skin flaps

Skin flap necrosis is most commonly seen in the post auricular region as a result of the increased tension that is placed on skin flaps which results in decreased blood circulation. Necrosis can occur in any area usually secondary to haematoma formation or dissection that is too superficial. Again, the surgeon should be careful to leave an adequate amount of fatty subcutaneous tissue on the skin flap to maintain adequate blood supply.

If necrosis of the flap does occur, conservative therapy with a moist dressing and healing by secondary intention often will still result in a good cosmetic outcome. However, it is not uncommon for scar tissue and pigmentation problems to occur.

This is an appropriate point to discuss smoking, which many surgeons believe significantly impairs skin flap circulation. All patients are advised to refrain from smoking for a period of time before surgery and immediately after. Patients who smoke should be advised that they run the risk of increased complication with a loss of the flap and/ or areas of necrosis. This should be documented in the patient's chart. There are some surgeons who believe that smoking in general is a contraindication to this procedure if the patient is not willing to stop in order to have the best chance of a favourable outcome.

Facial nerve injury

A slight paresis of the facial muscles can sometimes be detected for up to 12 hours after surgery. This is most commonly caused by a prolonged action of the local anaesthetic agent or oedema of the nerve itself. Most of these conditions resolve spontaneously and true facial paralysis is rare if the surgeon follows the short flap technique. Various authors have reported rates ranging from 0.1% to 2.6% for facial nerve paralysis following rhytidectomy.

As discussed previously in the facial anatomy section of this chapter, the temporal and marginal mandibular facial nerve branches are most susceptible to injury because of their anatomic position. The temporal frontal branch follows a plain that extend 0.5cm below the tragus to 1.5cm above the lateral extent of the eyebrow. This nerve continues to become more superficial as it extends anteriorly. The surgeon must change the dissection plain when switching from the temporal forehead unit to the facial unit, if this change does not occur, this nerve may be severed. This nerve has a close proximity to the superficial temporal artery and vein. The nerve is therefore also vulnerable to injury during attempts at obtaining haemostasis when these vessels are transected.

The marginal mandibular nerve runs 1 to 3cm below the horizontal ramus of the mandible, and external to the facial nerve and vein. The nerve then creates an arc which sends branches to the four muscles that depress the lower lip. It is in this location that the nerve is most susceptible to injury.

Again, as with many other surgical procedures, careful attention to anatomy and dissection can help decrease complications. The use of bipolar cautery is recommended for haemostatic control as well as reducing possible nerve injury.

If transection of the nerve is noted during the surgical procedure, primary repair should be attempted. This of course is not the usual case and secondary repair of these nerve branches is usually less than ideal because of the rather small calibre.

Skin flap perforation or button hole

If the skin flap is accidentally perforated, repair should be done immediately to avoid any further extension. A primary closure in two or three layers is recommended. If done properly, this area usually heals quite well.

Earlobe distortion

The commonly seen pulled or stretched earlobe will result in a cosmetically displeasing distortion. This is avoided by preventing excessive downward traction on the earlobe during flap recontouring. This situation may resolve post-operatively and no immediate repair is necessary.

If after to 6 to 12 months, there is still significant distortion, a correction with a small Z-plasty may help.

Alopecia

Alopecia following rhytidectomy is most commonly seen in the temporal region. Most of these cases will resolve spontaneously, but slowly. Hair growth is often slow and takes some time to camouflage this area. Alopecia can be avoided by careful attention to making incisions in the direction of the hair follicles. Overuse of cautery in the incision line will also destroy hair follicles as will excessive tension on the wound edge.

Hypertrophic scars

Hypertrophic or keloid scarring can occur in association with any surgery. Some of this may be predicted pre-operatively by taking a careful history from the patient. Hypertrophic scarring can also occur as a result of infection or skin flap necrosis with secondary healing. Flap closure under excessive tension should be avoided in all rhytidectomy patients. Most surgical scars are hidden behind the hairline and treatment is only necessary for the most excessive scars. Intralesional steroid injection may be utilised to help reduce scar formation. In only a rare number of cases, a surgical resection of the hypertrophic scar would be necessary. A change in the frontal hairline is a normal occurrence and consequence of a forehead lift. Placement of incisions more anteriorly can help preserve the preauricular temporal hair tuft. This may allow the patient the ability to camouflage the procedure with different types of hairstyles.

Rhytidectomy: a summary

Carefully planned and properly placed surgical incisions combined with a minimum elevation and SMAS plication technique can give the patient back their youthful appearance with minimal risk of complication or a downtime. Appropriate patient selection and pre-operative consultation is important as with any cosmetic procedure. The patient who is not willing to participate in their own care by stopping problematic medications or smoking is at an increased risk for problems and may not be a candidate for surgery.

As always, patient safety is the primary concern and to err on the side of conservatism can be the difference between a happy patient and a disastrous outcome. Remember, new materials and secondary procedures a few years down the line can always bring additional improvement without risking complication.

Otoplasty

Anatomy

The auricle or pinna diverges from the side of the head at an angle of approximately 30 degrees. The auricle consists of an elastic cartilage shell and thin integument, which is more closely adherent on the lateral aspect than on the medical aspect. The helical border terminates anteriorly in the crus, which lies almost horizontally above the external auditory canal meatus. The antihelix crowning the posterior conchal wall diverges into superior and inferior crura enclosing the triangular fossa. Between the helix and antihelix lies a long deep furrow, the scapha. The conchal cavity is composed of a cymba and cavum which arises from the floor and reaches the depth of approximately 1cm overlying the tragus and antitragus.

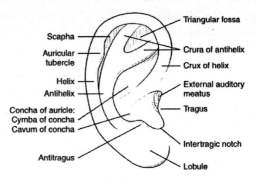

Anatomy of the normal auricle

Figure 4.32 Pinna anatomy

The blood supply is derived from the superficial, temporal and posterior auricular arteries. The sensory nerve supply is mainly from the anterior and posterior branches of the greater auricular nerve with somewhat lesser contributions from the auriculotemporal and lesser occipital nerves. This last fact is important when utilising a local anaesthesia block. Anesthetising the ear for surgical correction is easily accomplished by injecting anaesthetic along its base anteriorly and posteriorly.

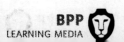

Embryology

In this section, we are concerned with the embryology primarily of the external ear and how it relates to congenital abnormalities including 'a prominent ear'. The external ear develops from the first branchial cleft and from portions of the adjacent first (mandibular) and second (hyoid) arches. At the end of the second month, the ectoderm moves inward forming a funnel shaped depression, which eventually evolves into the primary meatus and is connected to the expanding tympanic cavity by a solid strand of epithelial cells known as a meatal plate. At approximately the seventh month of development, a lumen develops, which becomes the osseous portion of the external auditory canal. The tympanic membrane is formed by a thinned out diaphragm of mesoderm lying between this external auditory canal and tympanic or middle ear cavity.

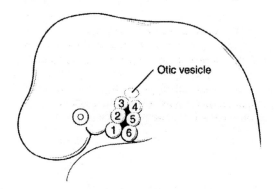

Figure 4.33 Hillocks of His in embryo

The auricle is formed from the six hillocks of His which first appear in the five-week embryo centred around the first branchial cleft. There are three on the posterior border of the first arch and three on the anterior border of the second arch. The exact relationship of these hillocks to specific structures is uncertain, but it is felt that the major portion of the auricle has its origin in the hyoid arch. The first and sixth hillocks maintain a fairly constant position, which marks the site of the developing tragus and antitragus respectively. The fourth and fifth tubercles expand and rotate across the dorsal end of the cleft, giving rise to the anterior helix and crus helicis as well as the body of the auricle. The growth of the mandibular arches depresses and probably contributes to the formation of the tragus.

Developmental abnormalities of the auricle and the correction of prominent ear

This common abnormality often creates a psychological rather than physical handicap. Correction should be undertaken prior to the child becoming the object of ridicule, which is often at approximately five years of age when they are about to enter school.

The pathology of this deformity is secondary to the development of the ear during gestation. During the third month, the auricle undergoes increasing protrusions in the side of the head at the end of the six-month margin of the helix has curled and the body of the antihelix has become definitely folded and the crura appear. Interference with the normal evolution of this process of folding produces prominent ears. If the usual prominent ear deformity stems from a failure of folding of the antihelix, which widens the scaphoconchal angle, this angle sometimes reaches 150 degrees or more with flattening of the superior crus. To a lesser extent, there may be flattening of the inferior crus as well.

Treatment

The surgical correction of the protruding ear has undergone many stages of development over the past 100 years or so.

1.   Dieffenbach (1845) described a simple excision of the skin from the auriculocephalic sulcus combined with sutures of the ear cartilage to the periosteum.

2.   Excision of conchal cartilage by Lelly (1888), Keen (1890), Monks (1981), and Cocherio (1894), all recognised the necessity of incising or excising a strip of the conchal wall. In addition to this, skin was also removed in order to produce a permanent change of the ear position. The popularity of this procedure is credited to Morestin in 1903.

3. Restoration of the antihelical fold by Luckett (1910): he was the first to emphasise the important concept that the deformity was essentially a failure of folding of the antihelix. He produced a permanent alteration of concha moving a long crescent of skin and cartilage extending almost the entire length of the ear.

4. Necessity of reducing the sharpness of the antihelix: there have been many attempts to eliminate the sharp antihelical outline produced by the initial Luckett procedure including the use of multiple parallel incisions. Becker (1949, 1952) improved over this method by omitting the Luckett incision and rolling in the delaminated borders of the antihelix to produce a cornucopia-like structure. This most closely resembled the normal superior crus. This method was further refined by Converse in 1955 and 1963. Converse omitted any incisions of the cartilage along the crest of the antihelix. To thin the cartilage, where necessary he used dermabrasive brushes and rolled the entire antihelix and crus into a single cornucopia.

A modification of this technique can work quite well and produce desirable results without any sharp edges and decreased chance of the cartilage cracking or fracturing. By removing skin and a portion of the perichondrium posteriorly to allow healing and scarring of the edges together, the antihelical fold can be reconstructed and held in position with nonabsorbable sutures while still giving a smooth natural contour (modified method of Mustarde).

Complications

Regardless of the otoplasty method employed, under-correction or recurrent deformity is always a potential problem. When properly performed, the method described above gives a normal auricular appearance, which is free of sharp antihelical edges and a flat scapha, which characterised the Luckett type procedure. Failure to introduce this efficient curve in the outline of the superior crus may give an unnatural straight appearance to the crus. Attention to haemostasis is important to prevent haematoma formation. This does not appear to be a significant problem in this procedure and no drains have been required post-operatively. A proper post-operative dressing with a packing in the crus of the auricle at the end of the procedure will help prevent any distortion of the mobilised cartilage. It should be noted that even though the cartilage has not been removed or cut, there is sufficient scarring within the tubed or folded portion to produce a permanent setback position.

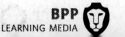

References

Arey, LB. (1984) *Developmental Anatomy. A Text Book and Laboratory Manual of Embryology.* 6th edition. Philadelphia: WB Saunders Company.

Baker, D and Conley, J. Avoiding the facial nerve injury and rhytidectomy. *Plastic and Reconstructive Surgery* 1979; 64 (6): 781.

Benson WH and McCullough, EG (1986) *Aesthetic Surgery of the Aging Face.* St. Louis-Toronto: CV Mosby Company.

Crysdale WS and Patham B. External septorhinoplasty in children. *Laryngoscope* 1985; 95: 12-16.

Converse JM (1968) *Reconstructive Plastic Surgery.* Philadelphia and London: WB Saunders Company Volume 3, pp. 1076–1077.

Goodman WS and Charbonneau PA. External approach to rhinoplasty. *Laryngoscope* 1974; 84: 2195-2201.

Goodman WS and Miller R. Surgery of the nasal tip by external rhinoplasty. *Ear, Nose, Throat,* 1982; J 61: 23-33.

His, W. Zur Entwicklungsgeschichte des Acustico – Facialgebietes beim Menschen. *Arch Anat Entwicklungsgesch.* 1889; 1–28

Livio M (2002) *The Golden Ratio.* New York: Broadway Books.

Mustarde JC. The treatment prominity by buried mattress sutures: 10-ERV survey. *Plastic Reconstruct Surg.* 1967; 39:3382.

Mustarde JC. The correction of prominent ears using simple mattress sutures. *Br J Plastic Surg.* 1963; 16:170.

Powell N and Humphries B (1984) *Proportions of the Aesthetic Face.* New York: Thieme-Stratton.

Rees, TD (1980) *Aesthetic Plastic Surgery Vol II,* Philadelphia: WB Saunders Company.

Ridley, MD and Van Hook SM (2002) 'Aesthetic facial proportions'. In Papel ID, ed. *Facial Plastic and Reconstructive Surgery.* New York-Stuttgard: Thieme. pp. 96-109.

Romm, S. (1992) *The Changing Face of Beauty.* St. Louis: Mosby-Yearbook.

Shikowitz MJ, Zahtz GD, and Goldstein MN. External rhinoplasty approach for malignant tumors of the anterior nasal septum. *American Journal of Rhinology* 1987; Summer 103-108.

Stone JW. External rhinoplasty. *Laryngoscope* 1980; 90: 1626–1630.

Tardy ME and Behrbohm H (2004) *The Essentials of Septorhinoplasty.* New York: Thieme.

Wright WK and Kridel RW. External septorhinoplasty; the tool for teaching and for improved results. *Laryngoscope* 1981; 91: 945-951.

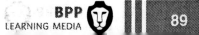

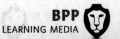

Practice questions

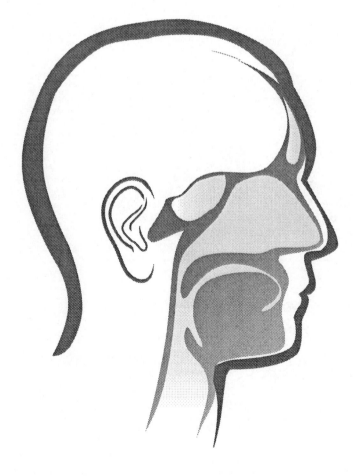

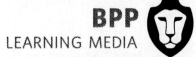
BPP LEARNING MEDIA

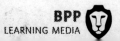

Otology

1. A 30-year-old woman presented with a six-month history of gradual onset right-sided hearing loss. On examination the ears are otoscopically normal. She is unable to hear a whispered voice 6 centimetres from the right ear but can do so on the left. On testing with a 512Hz tuning fork, bone conduction is better than air conduction for the right ear but not the left and the Weber response lateralises to the right ear.

    Which of the following best describe the location of the pathology responsible for her hearing loss?

    Scala Media

    Incus

    Round window

    Endolymphatic duct

    Stapes

2. A 45-year-old woman presented with a six-month history of gradual onset bilateral hearing loss. On examination the ears are otoscopically normal. She is unable to hear a whispered voice 6 centimetres in either ear. On testing with a 512Hz tuning fork, bone conduction is better than air conduction in both ears and the Weber response is equivocal.

    What is the most likely diagnosis?

    Otosclerosis

    Otitis media with effusion

    Presbyacusis

    Noise induced hearing loss

    Chronic Otitis Media

3. A 57-year-old lorry driver presented with a one-year history of gradually increasing left-sided hearing loss and tinnitus. On examination both tympanic membranes are normal. He is unable to hear conversational level voice presented at 6 centimetres from the left ear but can repeat whispered speech presented at the same distance in the right ear. Pure tone audiometery is consistent with a severe sensorineural hearing loss in the right ear.

    What is the most likely diagnosis?

    Labyrinthitis

    Otosclerosis

    Vestibular schwannoma

    Méniére's disease

    Presbyacusis

4. A 57-year-old lorry driver presented with a one-year history of gradually increasing left-sided hearing loss and tinnitus. On examination both tympanic membranes are normal. He is unable to hear conversational level voice presented at 6 centimetres from the left ear but can repeat whispered speech presented at the same distance in the right ear. Pure tone audiometery is consistent with a severe sensorineural hearing loss in the right ear.

    Which of the following tests is most likely to be diagnostic?

    Electrocochleogram

    Electroencephalogram

    Lateral skull X-ray

    CT head scan

    MRI head scan

5. A 60-year-old woman presented with a three-month history of repeated episodes of vertigo. The attacks last for one minute at a time and are triggered by rolling over in bed or looking up.

    What is the most likely diagnosis?

    Méniére's disease

    Vertebrobasilar ischemia

    Benign Paroxysmal Positional Vertigo

    Labyrinthitis

    Migraine

6. A 60-year-old woman presented with a three-month history of repeated episodes of vertigo. The attacks last for one minute at a time and are triggered by rolling over in bed or looking up.

    What is the most likely site of her pathology?

    Scala Media

    Superior semicircular canal

    Posterior semicircular canal

    Endolymphatic duct

    Vestibular nerve

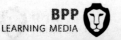

Rhinology

7. A 33-year-old man presents with a one-year history of a reduced sense of smell. He reports that he can still smell strong odours such as onions and bleach though they seem different to how he perceived them before. He does not have rhinorrohea or nasal obstruction.

    What is the most likely diagnosis?

    Nasal septal deviation

    Nasal polyps

    Perennial rhinitis

    Rhinitis medicamentosa

    Olfactory neuroblastoma

8. A 25-year-old woman presents with a four-month history of hyposmia following an upper respiratory tract infection. She has ongoing rhinorrhoea and nasal obstruction.

    What is the most likely diagnosis?

    Nasal septal deviation

    Nasal polyps

    Perennial rhinitis

    Rhinitis medicamentosa

    Olfactory neuroblastoma

9. Options

    A   Allergic rhinitis

    B   Vasomotor rhinitis

    C   Perennial rhinitis

    D   Cystic fibrosis

    E   Acute Rhinosinusitis

    F   Chronic Rhinosinusitis

    G   Viral rhinitis

    H   Rhinitis medicamentosa

    I   CSF rhinorrhoea

    J   Nasal foreign body

    For each of the clinical scenarios listed below, select the most appropriate diagnosis from the above list. Each of the listed options may be used once, more than once or not at all.

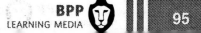

1. A 20-year-old woman presented in June with a two-month history of bilateral clear rhinorrhoea and sneezing worse on mornings. She does not smoke but is a well controlled asthmatic. On examination the nasal airway is restricted bilaterally. The nasal mucosa is oedematous and inflamed.

2. A 30-year-old builder presented with a four-month history of bilateral clear rhinorrhoea and nasal obstruction worse at night that persisted after a head cold he contracted in February. He gets relief with an over the counter topical nasal spray that he now uses four or more times a day. On examination the nasal airway is restricted bilaterally. The nasal mucosa is oedematous and inflamed.

3. An 18-year-old man with Down's syndrome presented with a three-month history of left nasal discharge. On examination there is purulent discharge in the left naris, the right is clear.

4. A 35-year-old obese woman presented with a two-month history of intermittent clear right nasal discharge. She does not smoke and has had no improvement with the use of topical nasal steroids. Anterior rhinoscopy was normal.

10. Epistaxis

A   Allergic rhinitis

B   Trauma

C   Anticoagulant medication

D   Foreign body

E   Neoplasm

F   Hereditary haemorrhagic telangiectasia

G   Nasal surgery

H   Cocaine abuse

I   Nasal vestibulitis

J   Coagulopathy

For each of the clinical scenarios listed below, select the most appropriate diagnosis from the above list. Each of the listed options may be used once, more than once or not at all.

1. A 92-year-old male presents to casualty with a two-hour history of epistaxis. Four weeks ago he had a thoracotomy and placement of a metallic mitral valve.

2. A five-year-old boy presents with left sided epistaxis. His parents report offensive smelling discharge from the same nostril for the last week, which has not responded to antibiotics from the general practitioner. On examination his left nostril shows inflamed mucosa with blood stained mucopurulent discharge.

3. A 35-year-old male presents to casualty following a bar room fight with a deviated septum and right sided epistaxis.

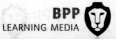

4. An elderly lady presents to the respiratory physicians with breathlessness on the background of recurrent and heavy epistaxis. On examination she has multiple red spots on her lips and cutaneous spots on her cheeks that under magnification appear to be capillaries. Body scanning subsequently revealed multiple liver and lung arteriovenous malformations.

11. Nasal blockage

    A   Deviated nasal bones

    B   Foreign bodies

    C   Deviated nasal septum

    D   Nasal polyps

    E   Rhinitis medicamentosa

    F   Wegener's granulomatosis

    G   Nasopharyngeal carcinoma

    H   Perennial allergic rhinitis

    I   Vasomotor rhinitis

    J   Viral rhinitis

For each of the clinical scenarios listed below, select the most appropriate diagnosis from the above list. Each of the listed options may be used once, more than once or not at all.

1. A 30-year-old woman presents with episodes of recurrent sneezing, watery rhinorrhoea and nasal blockage throughout the year. Her symptoms are worse at night.

2. A two-year-old child presents with a one-week history of an offensive unilateral nasal discharge.

3. An 18-year-old man, who suffered nasal trauma, complains of a persistent right-sided nasal obstruction for four months following the assault.

4. A 40-year-old man presents with a history of bilateral nasal blockage. He has temporary relief with an 'over-the-counter' decongestant that he has been using for the last two months.

Laryngology

12. Select the muscle innervated by the external laryngeal nerve.

Thyroarytenoid

Posterior cricoarytenoid

Thyrohyoid

Cricopharyngeus

Cricothyroid

13. The recurrent laryngeal nerve supplies which of the following muscles?

     Palatoglossus

     Interarytenoid

     Cricothyroid

     Omohyoid

     Sternothyroid

14. Options

     A   Upper respiratory tract infection

     B   Laryngitis

     C   Voice overuse

     D   Pharyngeal acid reflux

     E   Laryngeal carcinoma

     F   Trauma

     G   Hypothyroidism

     H   Laryngeal nerve palsy

     I   Motor neurone disease (MND)

     J   Myasthenia gravis

     For each of the clinical scenarios listed below, select the most appropriate diagnosis from the above list. Each of the listed options may be used once, more than once or not at all.

     1.   A 36-year-old female teacher is seen on the ward round the day following thyroid lobectomy and is noted to have developed a weak, breathy voice.

     2.   A 68-year-old retired long distance lorry driver who has smokes 15 cigarettes a day presents to the emergency department with breathlessness and a hoarse voice.

     3.   A 22-year-old trainee primary school teacher has been experiencing episodes of throat pain on speaking and a weak voice.

     4.   A 49-year-old business executive with a Basal Metabolic Index of 32 complains of a feeling of tightness in the throat and an intermittently hoarse voice but no dysphagia.

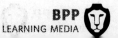

15. Options

    A   Rhinovirus

    B   Epstein-Barr virus

    C   Influenza virus

    D   HIV

    E   Beta haemolytic Streptococcus

    F   Candida albicans

    G   Staphyococcus aureus

    H   Haemophillus influenza

    I   Streptococcus pnuemoniae

For each of the clinical scenarios listed below, select the most appropriate causative organism from the above list. Each of the listed options may be used once, more than once or not at all.

1.   An 18-year-old university student is seen in the emergency department with a two-day history of fever, increasing sore throat and dysphagia. On examination the tonsils are symmetrically enlarged with an exudate over the surfaces and there are multiple palpable cervical lymph nodes.

2.   A 22-year-old teacher who has just completed a course of antibiotics for a urinary tract infection presents with a two-day history of odynophagia. On examination the pharynx is inflamed and the dorsum of the tongue is covered by a white membrane.

3.   A 35-year-old actor has been suffering from recurrent fever, sore throat and weight loss over the last six months. On examination there is an elevated bluish swelling on the hard palate and multiple cervical lymph nodes.

4.   A 15-year-old secondary school student has a four-day history of sore throat, loss of appetite and fever. On examination the tonsils are symmetrically enlarged with punctuate membrane. The jugulodigastric nodes are bilaterally enlarged. This is the third episode in six months.

16. Hoarseness of voice

    A   Acute laryngitis

    B   Chronic laryngitis

    C   Laryngeal carcinoma

    D   Sicca syndrome

    E   Hypothyroidism

    F   Singer's nodules

    G   Vocal cord palsy

    H   Laryngeal candidiasis

    I   Oesophageal carcinoma

    J   Bronchogenic carcinoma

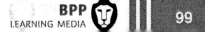

For each of the clinical scenarios listed below, select the most appropriate diagnosis from the above list. Each of the listed options may be used once, more than once or not at all.

1. A 24-year-old rock star presents to his GP with a six-week history of a hoarse voice. He had no dysphagia or odynophagia and denies any sore throat.

2. A 60-year-old heavy smoker and publican presented with a four-week history of hoarseness of voice. On mirror examination of the larynx there is a large white mass on the left vocal cord.

3. A 56-year-old woman complains of a hoarse voice following thyroid surgery.

4. A 65-year-old male following a renal transplant complains of being hoarse for many weeks. On examination his throat is red with white patches. The larynx and his vocal cords are red and inflamed. The cords move normally. He is on immunosuppression following his transplant.

Facial plastic surgery

17. When assessing facial symmetry, the face is usually divided by imaginary vertical lines such that the horizontal dimensions of the units are equal. Similarly imaginary horizontal lines can be used to divide the face into units of equal vertical dimension. How many vertical and horizontal units are there?

    A   4 vertical and 4 horizontal

    B   3 vertical and 4 horizontal

    C   4 vertical and 3 horizontal

    D   3 vertical and 5 horizontal

    E   5 vertical and 3 horizontal

18. Which of the following facial muscles is supplied by the marginal mandibular branch of the facial nerve?

    Levator labii superioris

    Procerous

    Depressor anguli oris

    Orbicularis oculi

    Buccinator

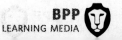

19. Facial anatomy

    A   Rhinion

    B   Nasion

    C   Tip defining point

    D   Trichion

    E   Subnasale

    F   Menton

    G   Pogonion

    H   Gnathion

    I   Cervical point

For each of the descriptions below select the most appropriate term from the list of options. Each of the listed options may be used once, more than once or not at all.

1. The junction of the hair bearing with the non-hair bearing forehead.
2. The most superior point of the nose, where it meets the forehead.
3. The junction of the nasal bone and quadrilateral septal cartilage.
4. The junction of the neck with the face.

20. Facial anatomy

    A   Skin flap necrosis

    B   Corneal ulceration

    C   Blindness

    D   Facial paralysis

    E   Alopecia

    F   Wound dehiscence

    G   Recurrent/residual deformity

    H   Wound infection

    I   Scarring

Select from one of the above listed options the one that best describes the most debilitating potential complication of each of the following surgical procedures. Each of the listed options may be used once, more than once or not at all.

1. A non-smoking 36-year-old female teacher is being counselled for open structure rhinoplasty.
2. A 60-year-old male office worker wishes to undergo rhytidectomy.
3. An 18-year-old male university student wants to have asymmetry of the pinna corrected.
4. A 49-year-old female business executive is being considered for blepharoplasty.

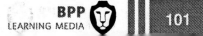

21. Post-operative complications of blepharoplasty

   A   Keratoconjunctivitis sicca

   B   Corneal ulcers

   C   Blindness

   D   Oedema

   E   Malignant hyperpyrexia

   F   Wound breakdown

   G   Haematoma

   H   Keloid scarring

   I   Cysts

   J   Post-operative nausea and vomiting

   For each of the clinical scenarios listed below, select the most appropriate diagnosis from the above list. Each of the listed options may be used once, more than once or not at all.

   1.   Two days following blepharoplasty a 42-year-old executive notices the wound coming apart and oozing from the base.

   2.   After waking up from the procedure a 54-year-old lady is troubled by persistent nausea and vomiting.

   3.   A 32-year-old African-American lady notices thickening of her scars.

   4.   A 60-year-old female complains of dry eyes following surgery.

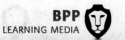

Answers to
practice questions

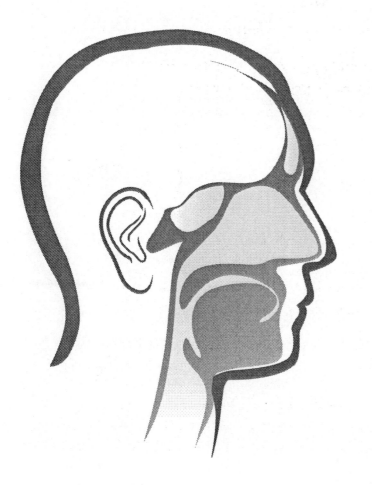

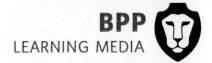

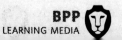

1.   Stapes

2.   Otosclerosis

3.   Vestibular schwannoma

4.   MRI head scan

5.   Benign paroxsysmal positional vertigo

6.   Posterior semicircular canal

7.   Olfactory neuroblastoma

8.   Perennial rhinitis

9.   9.1   A
        9.2   H
        9.3   J
        9.4   I

10.   10.1   C
        10.2   D
        10.3   B
        10.4   F

11.   11.1   H
        11.2   B
        11.3   C
        11.4   E

12.   Cricothyroid

13.   Interarytenoid

14.   14.1   H
        14.2   E
        14.3   C
        14.4   D

15.   15.1   B
        15.2   F
        15.3   D
        15.4   E

16.   15.1   F
        15.2   C
        15.3   G
        15.4   H

17.   E   5 vertical and 3 horizontal

18.   Depressor anguli oris

19.   19.1   D
        19.2   B
        19.3   A
        19.4   I

20.   20.1   I
       20.2   D
       20.3   G
       20.4   C

21.   21.1   E
       21.2   J
       21.3   H
       21.4   A

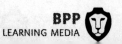

Index

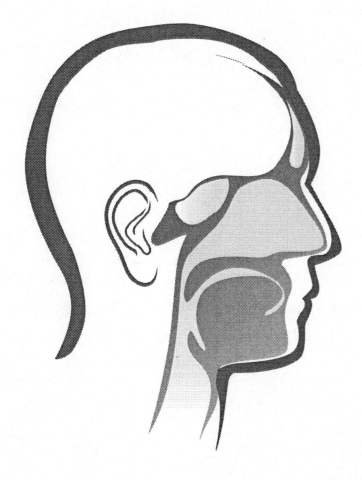

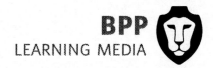

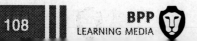

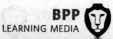

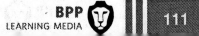

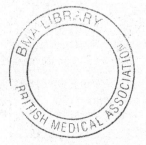

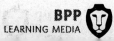